THE PHYSICIAN'S GUIDE TO

CATARACTS,

GLAUCOMA,

AND

OTHER

EYE PROBLEMS

THE PHYSICIAN'S GUIDE TO

◇

CATARACTS,

GLAUCOMA,

AND

OTHER

EYE PROBLEMS

◇

John Eden, M.D.,
and the Editors of
CONSUMER REPORTS BOOKS

CONSUMER REPORTS BOOKS
A Division of Consumers Union
Yonkers, New York

Copyright © 1992 by John Eden

Published by
Consumers Union of United States, Inc.,
Yonkers, New York 10703.
Some of the material in this book appeared previously in *The Eye Book* by John Eden,
copyright © 1978 by John Eden, published by The Viking Press, 375 Hudson St.,
New York, New York 10014.

Library of Congress Cataloging-in-Publication Data
Eden, John, 1933–
The physician's guide to cataracts, glaucoma, and other eye
problems / by John Eden and the editors of Consumer Reports Books ;
[illustrations by Laszlo Kubinyi].
p.   cm.
ISBN 0-89043-425-5
1. Eye—Diseases and defects.   2. Cataract.   3. Glaucoma.
I. Consumer Reports Books.   II. Title.
RE46.E32   1991
617.7'1—dc20   92-7413
                                                                 CIP

Design by GDS/Jeffrey L. Ward
Illustrations by Laszlo Kubinyi
First printing, May 1992
Manufactured in the United States of America

To Bob

Contents

Introduction 1
1. How We See 3
2. The Routine Eye Examination 21
3. The Optical Errors: Nearsightedness, Farsightedness, Astigmatism, and Presbyopia 42
4. Correcting Optical Errors: Eyeglasses and Contact Lenses 58
5. About Cataracts 106
6. If You Have a Cataract 114
7. About Glaucoma 147
8. If You Have Glaucoma 170
9. Other Common Diseases of the Eye 195
10. Commonsense Eye Care: How to Spend the Least to Get the Best 223
    Glossary 273
    Appendix: Useful Addresses 305
    Index 307

Introduction

◇

Now living in Sagaponack, New York—after having spent over twenty-five years in private ophthalmology practice in Manhattan and having written a book on eyes and eye care over ten years ago that had made its way into three foreign editions—I thought it was a good time to write *The Physician's Guide to Cataracts, Glaucoma, and Other Eye Problems,* which is directed primarily at readers over age 40 and concerned members of their families. The book therefore emphasizes eye problems most often encountered after the onset of middle age, an area of knowledge where what you don't know can surely hurt you.

Less than 100 years ago, two diseases of the eye—cataracts and glaucoma—were among the most feared scourges of advancing age because they almost always led to blindness. Now the sight that is lost to cataracts can be recovered, and the damage caused by glaucoma can be prevented through early diagnosis and treatment. But in both cases this can be accomplished only if you seek the medical help available to you.

Cataracts remain an almost universal problem among those lucky enough to live a long life and account for nearly one million operations in the United States each year. The vast majority of these operations provide the cataract patient with an almost miraculous return of vision. Glaucoma strikes one in 25 people over the age of 40. Because of the insidiously silent course it takes—and public ignorance of the threat it poses—this disease continues to be a major cause of blindness. This is true despite the fact that blindness resulting from glaucoma is almost completely preventable if ophthalmic checkups are regularly performed on people over age 40.

Readers will also find information about glasses and contact lenses, eye infections, and major eye diseases that strike people of all ages. They will discover sound advice on practical eye care and a full discussion of economic considerations ranging from money-saving tips on eye medications to such issues as getting second opinions, understanding the ins and outs of medical insurance, and avoiding unnecessary medical procedures.

Unfortunately, many well-established myths deter the general public from a better understanding of how we see and what we can do to protect this most important of the five senses. It is my hope that by demystifying the eye and explaining in simple terms how this wonderful organ works and what can go wrong with it, I will have made it possible for readers of this book to care for their eyes more intelligently and more economically.

How We See

◇

MYTH: Babies can see at birth.
FACT: Although the eyes are anatomically developed at birth, we do not come into the world as seeing creatures. Newborn babies are aware of little more than the difference between light and dark. We must learn to see, just as we must learn to talk, and this learning process takes place gradually, between birth and age six.

MYTH: Contact lenses, or indeed any small foreign particles that get into our eyes, can work their way back behind the eyeball and get lost inside our head.
FACT: The exposed front of the eyeball is separated from the back portion by a membrane called the conjunctiva. This provides a barrier that makes it impossible for foreign bodies, such as particles of dust or contact lenses, to travel beyond the outer part of the eyeball to the inside of the head.

MYTH: Blue eyes are more delicate than brown eyes, and therefore are more susceptible to irritation and other eye problems.

FACT: The only difference between blue and brown eyes is in the amount of pigment in the iris. The pigment in the iris blocks the passage of light, and because blue eyes have less pigment than brown eyes, they may be somewhat more sensitive to light. But they are not otherwise more vulnerable to irritation or other eye problems.

Perhaps more than any one of our senses, sight establishes our contact with the world around us. Our ability to see the shape, size, and color of things, thereby determining where we stand in the scheme of things, is a gift of nature we tend to take for granted. Our eyes are remarkable instruments, perfectly designed to collect a wide range of bold and subtle visual information. Along with the brain, to which all this information is sent via a specialized nerve network for sorting and analysis, our eyes provide us with the vision we depend on so heavily.

Anatomy and Function of the Eyeball

The human eye is a dual organ—two eyes working together to transmit visual information to the brain. Although it is possible to see with a single eye, it takes two normally functioning eyes to provide the brain with all the visual information it can use.

The eye is made up of numerous kinds of highly specialized cells performing a variety of functions. The cells are arranged into the muscular, fibrous connective, circulatory, and nervous systems specific to the eye. Although these systems are similar to others serving different organs throughout the body, they are especially designed to aid the eye in doing its job.

The normal adult eyeball is an elliptical sphere, which means it is more egg-shaped than perfectly round. It has three distinct concentric layers of tissue. The first layer, which serves to protect your eye's delicate internal structures, consists of the *sclera,** the opaque white of the eye, and the *cornea,* the transparent layer that lies in front of the *pupil* and *iris.*

The sclera covers about five-sixths of the surface of the eyeball. It is interrupted only by the cornea in front, and the *optic nerve,* which enters the eyeball at the back. Although not much thicker than the page you are now reading, the cornea and sclera are composed of extremely tough tissues. While it is not impossible to pierce them, it would require a very sharp object traveling at high speed to do so.

A thin membrane called the *conjunctiva,* which is not technically a part of the eyeball, separates the exposed front and unexposed back portions of the eye. It covers the front part of the sclera and then laps over and continues forward onto the inner surface of the upper and lower eyelids. The conjunctiva thus closes off the back of the eyeball, making it impossible for dust particles or any other matter to get lost in your eye or travel back inside your head.

The second of the three layers is called the *uveal tract,* and its main functions are circulatory and muscular. The uveal tract itself consists of the iris, the *ciliary body,* and the *choroid.*

The iris is the round colored part of the eye that surrounds the pupil, and it is responsible for what we call eye

*Major terms defined in the glossary are italicized in the text the first time they are mentioned.

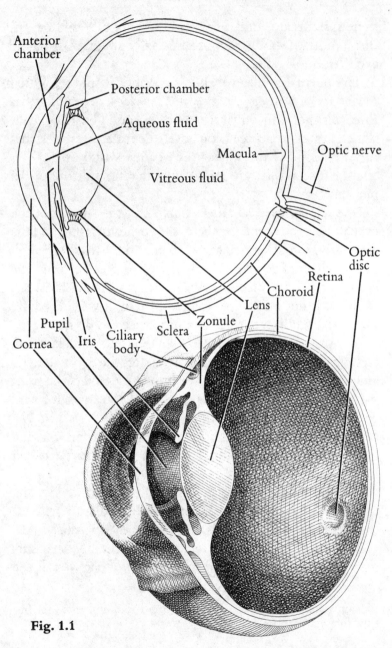

Fig. 1.1

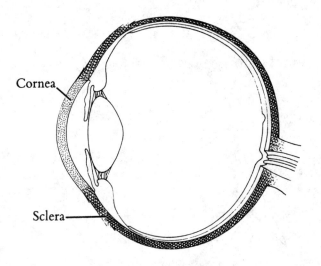

Fig. 1.2 The protective layer of the eyeball

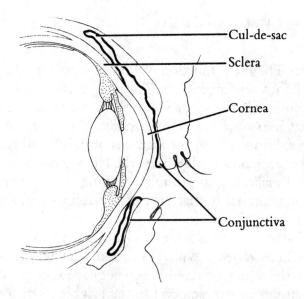

Fig. 1.3 The conjunctiva

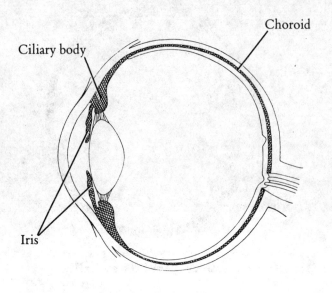

Fig. 1.4   The uveal tract

color. The main function of the iris is to permit more or less light to enter your eye. The pupil itself is simply a hole surrounded by the iris, and it is through this hole that light passes into your eye. The involuntary muscles of the iris respond primarily to the stimulus of light, constricting to make the pupil a smaller hole when light is bright and dilating to make it a larger hole when light is dimmer. This action is similar to that of the iris diaphragm in a camera, but not exactly.

The human iris is not a mechanical device whose opening can be varied at will. The action is involuntary. Moreover, the muscles of your iris do not have a limited number of settings that correspond to the brightness of the light. They are continuously adjusting and readjusting to the level of light, remaining stationary only when the level of light stays the same. They respond to all changes in light, no matter how subtle, and their adjustments are often minutely fine. For example, going from a darkened movie house to bright daylight is a dramatic change, but it is by no means the only sort of adjustment the iris can make.

The ciliary body lies between the iris and the choroid. Like the iris, its function is primarily muscular. It is connected at both ends of the lens by a ligament-like tissue called the *zonule,* from which the *lens* is suspended like a person lying in a hammock. The muscles of the ciliary body contract or relax to alter the shape of the lens, thereby changing the surface through which light rays must pass to be received by your eye. This allows your eye to focus for near vision, refocus on objects at a distance, and then focus once again on nearby objects.

When the brain tells the eye to bring an object into focus, these muscles bend the lens until the brain reports that the image is clear. Of course, this happens so quickly that if you have normally functioning eyes, you are totally unaware of the process. It seems that as soon as you look at any object, it is immediately in focus. These are the muscles that medical professionals refer to when they speak of the focusing muscles of the eye.

The ciliary body has a second function: to secrete *aqueous fluid,* a substance that is extracted from the blood that the choroid brings to the eye. It flows from the area between the lens and the iris (the *posterior chamber*) into the area between the iris and the cornea (the *anterior chamber*). The waste-laden fluid is then reabsorbed into the blood. This dynamic circulation assures that aqueous fluid is constantly secreted into and drained away from the eye.

Behind the ciliary body is the choroid, the main circu-

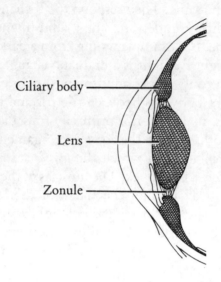

**Fig. 1.5   The structures that allow the eye to focus for
near vision.**

latory layer through which blood is carried to nourish the
various parts of the eye. This is not the eyeball's only blood
supply; the retina, for example, has its own circulatory system. Increasingly tiny arteries branch out from the choroid
to those portions of the eye that require blood, and the veins
carry blood laden with carbon dioxide and waste back to the
choroid. Some parts of the eye cannot be nourished in this
way because the presence of blood vessels would interfere
with their optical function. Nature has compensated for
this by providing other ways to supply oxygen to those tissues and carrying away waste in the aqueous fluid.

The innermost layer of the eye is the *retina,* an extremely
thin sheet of specialized nerve tissue made up of 10 distinct

cell layers, each of which performs a specific task in receiving visual images and transmitting them, via the optic nerve, to the brain. To go back to the camera analogy, the retina is like the film on which images are focused and recorded, but the retina is even more complicated and can function more effectively than film. The retina receives and passes along to the brain a very complex visual message, including the size, shape, dimension, position in space, relative distance, and color of an object.

The key central area of the retina, located slightly to the outer side of the eyeball, is called the *macula*. This tiny area, which represents about three percent of the total retina, is its most vital part. The macula is responsible for sharp central vision, and it is this area of the retina that permits nor-

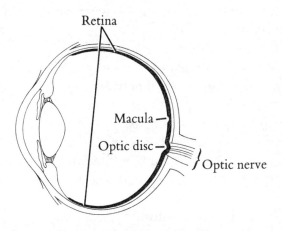

Fig. 1.6　The retina

mal 20/20 vision; the rest of the retina receives peripheral, or side, vision, and it delivers an image that is not as sharp as that coming from the macula.

Although blood vessels crisscross almost the entire retinal surface, the macula is one area that cannot be supplied directly in this way. Because its highly sensitive receptor cells would be obscured by blood vessels, small capillaries feed into the edge of the macula; the exchange of oxygen and carbon dioxide in the center actually takes place by absorption through cell walls. Nature's solution to the problem works quite well as long as nothing interferes with this delicate process, but it does make the macula more vulnerable to damage than the rest of the retina.

In addition to its receptor properties, the retina is able to adapt to light and darkness. The iris performs the task of admitting or excluding light from the interior of the eye, and certain cells of the retina—the *rods* and *cones*—undergo photochemical changes that enable you to see at various light levels. For example, when you go from the daylight outdoors into a dimly lit room, the rods are activated and the cones deactivated to adjust to the lower level of light; when you return to the sunlight, the cones are again activated and the rods deactivated. It takes some time for the retina to adjust to the light change—an hour for complete *light adaptation* or *dark adaptation,* although you will be able to see well in much less time. This is why a room can often seem quite dark for a while after you come inside on a sunny day. The cones are also responsible for your ability to perceive colors.

All the visual information collected and recorded by the eye is transmitted to the brain by the optic nerve, which enters the eye at the back of the retina. The lack of retinal tissue at this point results in a *blind spot,* a very small area that cannot receive visual messages. An eye doctor can locate and measure your blind spot by covering one of your eyes at a time and administering a special test. However, under normal conditions you will not notice the blind spot because the area you cannot see with one eye will be seen by the other eye.

The Passage of Visual Information

Imagine a ray of light passing directly from the retina to an object you are viewing. This imaginary line is called the *visual axis,* and it must run through a series of perfectly clear structures so that no light is lost and no distortion or obstruction of the image takes place. These clear structures are called the *optical media,* and they are, from the front to the back of the eye, the cornea, the aqueous fluid, the lens, and the *vitreous fluid.*

Like the macula, the cornea is not obstructed by blood vessels, which would interfere with optical clarity. The cornea's metabolism is provided from tears on the outside and aqueous fluid on the inside. Both of these liquids can carry oxygen and carbon dioxide, just as blood does, but they are clear, so light can pass through them. Tears are secreted onto the surface of the eyeball by *lacrimal glands,* which are located inside the bony eye socket and drained away through small passages located in the eyelids.

In addition to its protective function, the cornea acts as a refractive (light-bending) *surface* in the visual axis. It is the first curved structure that light hits, and it bends the angle of the light rays inward, narrowing the beam as it enters the eye.

From the cornea, the light travels through the aqueous

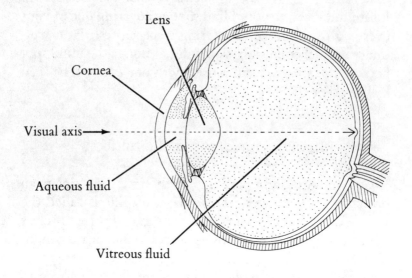

Fig. 1.7 The visual axis passes through the clear optical media.

fluid until it meets the lens, which bends it further. Though you can understand much about the lens by comparing it with various manufactured lenses, nature's lens is more complex and therefore much more effective. It is not a rigid piece of glass or plastic that must be moved forward or back to focus, but a flexible unit that can alter its shape to bring near or distant objects into focus. Like the cornea, the lens must be perfectly transparent. Therefore, it contains no blood vessels but instead receives its main nourishment from the aqueous fluid.

The lens grows throughout a person's life. As in a tree, new cell layers are produced on the outer surface in a continual concentric pattern. There is a slight increase in the size of the lens each time a layer is added, the layers becoming compressed with age and tending to become less elastic and, later in life, less clear.

Behind the lens, the eyeball is filled up with another optically clear substance, the vitreous fluid. Unlike the aqueous type, the vitreous is a stable gel-like mass that does not circulate and cannot be manufactured by the eye. Its function is mostly to maintain the shape and resilience of the eyeball and to provide a clear medium through which light can pass to the retina after having been bent by the lens.

Structural Protection

Each eyeball is suspended inside a cone-shaped skeletal socket called the *bony orbit,* which has a hole in the back through which run the optic nerve, the main blood vessels of the eye, and other nerves that serve the eye. The orbit protects the eyeball; the upper and lower ridges (the brow and cheekbone) are the first surfaces to receive the impact from a blow to the eye. Fatty and fibrous tissue surround the eyeball and serve to cushion it within the orbit. The upper and lower eyelids also protect the eye, and the eyelashes are an effective barrier against dust and other airborne bodies. In addition, the eyelids are lined with conjunctival membrane and contain the passages through which tears enter and drain from the eye to keep the exposed part of the eyeball nourished, lubricated, and smooth.

The inner eye muscles of the ciliary body are responsible for bending the lens, but there are also external muscles that control eye movement. Six main muscles in each eye perform this function, and they are paired to allow you to

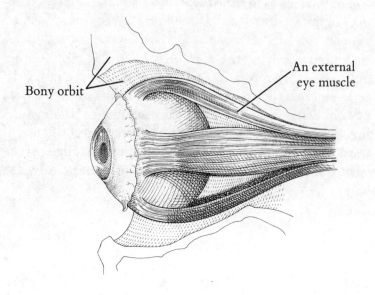

**Fig. 1.8   Eyeball in socket, showing three of the external
eye muscles**

move your eyes. These muscles are attached around the side
of the eyeball, behind the conjunctival barrier, and at the
back of the orbit.

The Visual Process

The various components of the human eye work in a
unique fashion to make vision possible. The camera resembles a simplified eye, but once the image has been recorded
on film, the camera's work is finished. A lab must develop
the film if anything is to be seen. In the human eye the

visual process has really just begun when rays of light reach the retina. The interpretation of visual data by the brain is a significant part of seeing. It is not enough to have two healthy eyes with all their working parts in order; we must also learn how to interpret the information that the eyes deliver to the brain.

We do not see at birth. We are not blind, but we simply have not learned to "read" the information brought to the brain by our eyes. Learning to make sense out of all this information takes place gradually during the first years of life, so we cannot say, for example, that at a certain age a child first learns to distinguish colors or at another age he or she is able to tell that one object is closer than another. From the moment we are born, our brain starts learning to use the message our eyes bring to it. It also sends messages back to the eyes about what additional kinds of information it would like to have. Over time our eyes develop the ability to transmit clearer and more refined images, and our brain learns to apply experience in guessing at what these images might mean.

In general, it is thought that nearly all this learning takes place between birth and age six. You may have observed that a young child can easily learn a new language well enough to speak it without an accent, but that as we grow older learning new languages becomes very much more difficult. In the same way, nature seems to have given children under the age of six a special ability to develop skill at perceiving size, color, shape, distance, spatial relations, and three dimensions. When abnormalities interfere with this learning process and go uncorrected until after age six, the development of normal vision skills becomes virtually impossible.

Recording an Image

In order to see a flower, for example, there must be light. You do not actually see objects; you see light reflected off objects, which is why you can see nothing at all in total darkness. The less light there is, the less clearly you will see. The retina will adapt and your iris will dilate or constrict according to the level of available light, but there must be at least some light present.

The air between the lighted flower and the front surface of the eye must be clear. You know that it is harder to see when it is foggy or when you look through a dirty windowpane, and that it is impossible to see at all if there is a solid object blocking the light directly in front of the thing you want to see.

If the light thrown off from the flower has traveled through unobstructed space, light rays will reach your cornea, where they are bent inward by its curved surface and transmitted through the aqueous fluid and onto the lens. At this point the lens bends the light rays further so they can then travel through the clear vitreous fluid and finally end their journey as a focused image on the surface of the retina. Because the retina is not optically clear, the light cannot travel any farther.

At this point the retina's image of the flower is upside down and flat. There is no mechanism within the eye to reverse it—no mirrors or prisms. The righting of the image is accomplished in the brain and is the result of a learned process.

Seeing objects as solid and three-dimensional is also something you must learn. True three-dimensional vision cannot exist if only one eye is doing the seeing or if your

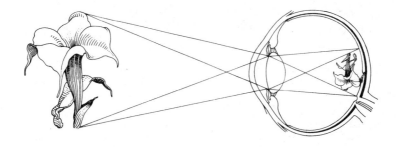

Fig. 1.9   A focused image arrives at the retina after traveling as rays of light through space and the clear optical media of the eye.

eyes are out of alignment and looking at different things. But even if your two eyes are aligned, a three-dimensional picture cannot be seen until the brain has learned to interpret the information it gets.

Visual data is transmitted by the *optic nerve* along a network that travels to the visual center of the brain. The message is in a sort of code that the brain has learned, and it contains information about the size, shape, and color of the objects. It also reports the specific part of the retina that received the image—a kind of return address. For example, an image received by the macula and recorded by the highly specialized macular cells will be received by the brain as a clear object viewed straight on. An image

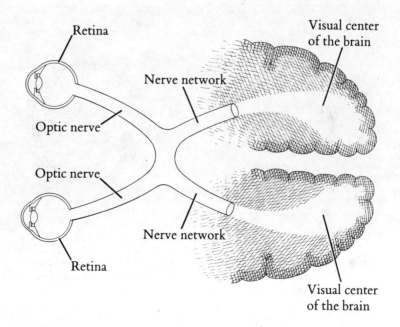

Fig. 1.10   The visual pathway to the brain

received by a peripheral part of the retina will arrive at the brain with data about its retinal origin, and the brain will "read" it as an object off to the left or right or wherever.

Our eyes and brain work together in this fashion to give us visual knowledge of the environment around us. Although it is vital to our sight that we be equipped with two structurally normal and healthy eyes, they alone will not permit us to see. Whereas the human eye is a perfectly designed collector of visual data, the human brain is the perfect decoder, and the partnership of the two is what gives us our highly sophisticated visual system.

The Routine Eye Examination

◇

MYTH: If you do not wear glasses, you do not have to have your eyes checked periodically.

FACT: Everyone should visit an eye doctor for regular eye checkups. People who do not wear corrective lenses can wait longer between appointments, but preventive medical examinations for total eye health, particularly past age 40, are as important for people without optical errors as they are for those who have them.

MYTH: If you give a wrong answer while your vision is being tested, you will end up with the wrong prescription for glasses or contact lenses.

FACT: The vision check has both a subjective element (based on patient response) and objective component (based on measurement with instruments). Any finding that differs significantly between the two will be rechecked. But the objective data can be used on their own to get a very accurate reading, as is the case with very young children and individuals who are mentally incapable of responding to the subjective portion of the checkup.

MYTH: During an eye exam a dilated pupil will cause your vision to be blurred.
FACT: Many people believe this is true, since one type of eyedrops an eye doctor may use to dilate the pupils also causes blurred vision. In fact, this temporary effect is caused by a component of these drops that paralyzes the near-focusing muscles. The loss of focusing ability, *not* the dilation of the pupils, is what causes the blur. Minimal visual irritation can be caused just by dilation.

There is an air of mystery about an eye examination that is absent from other periodic health checkups. When your physician thumps your knee with a rubber mallet, you know that he is checking your reflexes. You might not completely understand the mechanism of reflexes or know what a good or bad reflex indicates, but you do know that your reflex is what is being tested. When your dentist pokes around your mouth with a small metal probe, you know he is looking for cavities. But what is your ophthalmologist doing when he puts your chin on a platform in front of an instrument that looks like something out of NASA mission control? And why is the eye doctor shining a beam into your eyes? Why is the doctor asking you how many dots you see or whether a particular object is above or below a line? Why is the doctor putting eyedrops in your eyes, and why do the drops make it impossible for you to read a magazine while you wait for them to take effect? How, after all, can someone else tell what you see and whether or not you see it properly? More important, how can those simple exercises you are asked to perform during your examination tell your doctor if you have the first signs of a serious progressive disease, such as glaucoma, or if you are developing cataracts?

The examination described in this chapter is the routine preventive eye examination and does not include the more narrowly focused tests performed when some finding in the routine examination seems abnormal. If the routine exam suggests a possible problem, your doctor will do those additional tests that will give him or her information about the particular problem the doctor suspects. Although each ophthalmologist develops his or her own techniques for the routine examination, the similarities between doctors are greater than the differences.

Who Should Have an Eye Examination?

Everyone! Even if you do not wear glasses, even if you think you see well enough, a periodic eye checkup is an important part of your total program of preventive medicine—just like regular physical exams and visits to the dentist. As we grow older, our eyes and our visual needs change, and certain disorders may develop. Some, like glaucoma and cataracts, are specific to the eye; others, such as certain circulatory problems, often show up in the eye and can be diagnosed by your eye doctor. In early childhood the routine eye exam is of particularly great importance. Everyone's first visit to an ophthalmologist should occur at age three, when it is still possible to correct problems that might interfere with later visual development. If all is well, the next visit should be a preschool exam at age six. Those who wear corrective lenses should have their eyes examined about once every eighteen months after that. If your eyes need no correction, a checkup once every two or three years is sufficient until you reach your 40s. At that time you should increase your visits to once a year, whether or not you wear glasses or contact lenses, since this is the age when glaucoma is most likely to develop.

In the Consultation Room

Good examinations begin with a complete patient history. In order to treat you as an individual, the doctor needs to know certain details about the general state of your health, childhood diseases you have had, family medical history, and allergies to drugs or other substances. You have surely been asked a similar series of questions by your physician, but you may wonder why an eye doctor needs to know these things.

Many eye problems may be related to hereditary factors, so your family eye and medical history will tell the doctor whether or not there are any special signs to watch out for. Your doctor may need to prescribe medication, and he or she wants to be sure not to choose one to which you may be allergic. And finally, your eye health is related in many ways to your total physical health, and the more known about it, the better your doctor is able to look after your eyes.

After providing this general information, you will be asked a series of questions that zero in on your eyes. Have you had any eye ailments? Do you wear glasses? If so, how long have you worn them? How old is your current pair of glasses? How often do you wear your glasses—for reading only, for seeing far away only, or all the time? Do you wear contact lenses? When did you first get them, and when were they last checked? Do you experience any particular discomfort or difficulty with them? Is there any family history of glaucoma or other eye disease?

Finally, and perhaps most important, your doctor should ask if you have any complaints. Although you may have made your appointment because it was time for a periodic checkup, many people are moved to see their eye doctors only when some problem has been troubling them, either consciously or unconsciously. Even if your doctor does not ask for specific complaints, do not pass up this opportunity to ask your questions and express your concerns. Even the most expert physician cannot possibly pick up on everything wrong with your vision in one periodic examination.

In the Examination Room

Up to this point it has all been talk. Now you will be taken into an examination room for a series of tests. In some of them the doctor will observe the results *(objective tests);* in others you will be asked to report what you see *(subjective tests)*. Some of the tests will take place in a darkened room, others in the light. For some tests your vision will be altered in certain ways; for others it will be left in its natural state. Your doctor will use a battery of instruments, a few of which are simple, everyday objects while others are very specialized. Most of the tests are designed to yield specific diagnostic information; a few others are screening tests, meaning that they are designed to alert the doctor to signs of possible trouble that should be investigated further.

Snellen Chart

For the first test, your doctor will likely ask you to read a *Snellen chart*—those familiar rows of letters that diminish in size from top to bottom. You will read selected lines of the chart aloud under various circumstances—with corrective lenses if you wear them—first with one eye covered and then the other. Then your near vision will be tested by having you read aloud from a page of text you are holding close up.

Lensometer

If you wear glasses, you will be asked to produce them so that the prescription can be recorded and then compared to the findings obtained in the examination. The doctor ascertains the exact prescription of your glasses by looking at them through an instrument called a *lensometer,* which "reads" off the full prescription of each lens. Some offices

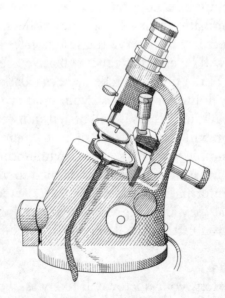

Fig. 2.1   A type of lensometer

possess a computerized lensometer, which can be operated by a technician and produces a printout of the prescription.

Physical Exam

The next step is a physical examination of your eyes, starting from the outside to look at the overall anatomy of the eye area—the eyebrows, eyelids, and eyelashes, in addition to the eyeball itself—to see if the area is symmetrical or if there are any growths, scars, redness, excessive tearing, or other signs of abnormality. Your eyelids will be pulled down and, with a penlight and magnifying lenses, the inner surface of the lids will be examined.

The doctor will focus on the eyeball itself to determine if your pupils react normally to light, if your eyeballs are reddened, or if there is any abnormal pigmentation or growth on the sclera or the conjunctiva. He or she will also confirm that the visible portion of your eyeball looks normal and that these various parts are in their proper position. If there are any abnormalities, the doctor will look further for causes, but at this point the doctor is mainly interested in the immediately obvious appearance of your eyes. Later the physician will make a very minute and detailed examination of both external and internal anatomy.

Eye-Muscle Tests

Next your eye-muscle balance will be checked to make sure that your eyes work together normally. The five tests commonly used to determine if the eye muscles are properly coordinated answer three basic questions: Can you move both eyes together in all directions? Can you keep your eyes parallel to each other on all planes? And do you see the same thing with each eye? The form the tests take and the instruments used may vary somewhat from one doctor to another, but they all yield the same information. Although these tests might need some explanation, each one takes less than five seconds.

The first test examines the external movement of your eyes. You will be asked to follow a penlight with both eyes as it is moved in a full circle within the periphery of your vision. Meanwhile, the physician will be watching your eyes to see if you can move them in all directions as far as you should, and if both eyes move together.

The second test requires that you wear a special pair of glasses with a red lens over the right eye and a green lens over the left. The doctor sits facing you and holds a flashlight that shines four small circular dots directly at you.

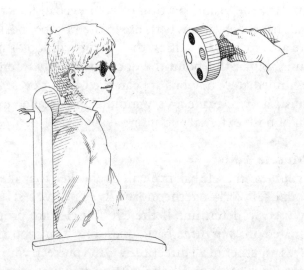

Fig. 2.2   The four-dot test, one of the basic tests for eye-muscle function

Two of the dots are red, one is green, and one is white. The combination of the colored lenses and the color of the various dots makes it possible for each eye to see some dots but not others. The doctor will ask you to look at the light with both eyes and report how many dots you see. There are four possible answers, all of which reveal whether or not you are using both eyes together and, if not, which eye you are using. If you say you see four dots, it means you are using both eyes and everything is normal. If you see two dots, you are using your left eye only; three dots means you are using your right eye only; and five dots indicates you have true double vision and are using both eyes but not simultaneously.

The next routine is a check of your vertical muscle balance to be sure that you can hold both eyes at the same level when you look at something. The doctor puts a special lens in front of one of your eyes and shines a penlight directly at you while you stare straight ahead and look out with both eyes. You will see a horizontal red line and a white spot of light, and you will then be asked to report whether the spot is above, below, or on the line. If you say it is on the line, your vertical balance is normal. If you see it *above or below* the line, you have a vertical misalignment. This is how the test works: The eye without the lens sees the spot of light from the penlight; the lens over the other eye turns that spot of light into a red line. Even though both eyes are looking right at the penlight, each eye sees something different. If the eyes are aligned, the eye behind the lens will be looking in exactly the same place as the other eye, and the spot and the line will appear to be in the same place. If the eyes are not aligned, however, the spot will appear to be above or below the line because both eyes will not be looking in the same place. Horizontal alignment can be tested by rotating the lens so the line is horizontal and the spot of light is seen either on the line or to the left or right of it.

The doctor then does an objective test that is very helpful because it can pick up even the subtlest degree of *strabismus,* commonly known as "cross-eye." He or she quickly covers and uncovers each of your eyes one at a time while you stare with both eyes at a penlight straight in front of you. The doctor watches the test eye to see if it jumps when he uncovers it. If it remains staring straight ahead, your eyes are properly aligned. If the eye moves in or out, this is evidence of strabismus, and further measurements must be done.

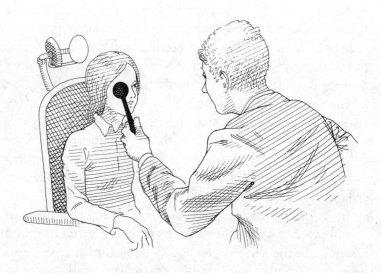

Fig. 2.3   The cover test, another of the basic tests for eye-muscle function

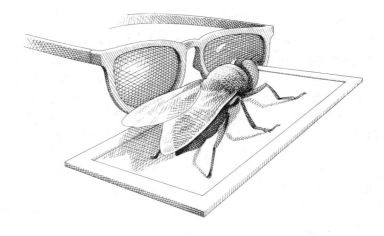

Fig. 2.4 **If you have normal, three-dimensional vision, this is how the picture of the fly will look to you.**

In the next test, you will be checked to see if you can use both eyes together to deliver a three-dimensional image to the brain. You will be asked to wear another pair of special glasses and look at a picture, usually of a fly, specially drawn so it will appear three-dimensional with the glasses if you have normal depth perception. If your depth perception is not normally developed, the fly will appear flat, even with the glasses.

At this point in the eye exam, the doctor knows how well you can see and whether there is any gross physical evidence of disease or structural abnormality. He also knows if you can move your eyes normally, how well they are coordinated, and whether or not you have normal depth perception.

Biomicroscope

Now it is time for a closer, more revealing look at the anatomy of your eyes. With the help of that window into your eye, the pupil, an eye doctor can do an internal examination without the use of X rays or exploratory surgery. The instrument he or she uses to do this is called a *biomicroscope*, or slit lamp. Some patients say that this instrument looks like a medieval torture device, but the exam the doctor performs with it is quite painless. You will be asked to put your chin on the biomicroscope's chin rest and keep staring straight ahead while the doctor shines various beams of light into your eyes.

The instrument is equipped with a powerful microscope that enlarges the tissues in the parts of the eye being examined. The light and lens system works in three ways to permit this minute examination. First, the very bright lights illuminate the darkened inside of your eye. Second, the magnification allows the doctor to see things too small to be observed with the naked eye. Third, the lamp focuses a narrow beam of light that, along with its lens, reveals an optically thin section of eye tissue that can then be examined much as a pathologist studies a slide of tissue under a conventional microscope. In this case, of course, the "slide" also consists of living tissue, which is why the instrument is called a *bio*-(living) microscope. This is a particularly valuable aid, since the actual removal of eye tissue for microscopic evaluation cannot be done without seriously injuring the eye.

Through the biomicroscope, the doctor can take a closer look at the parts of the eye that were examined in less detail

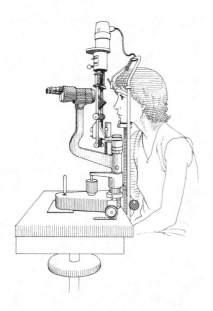

Fig. 2.5 Biomicroscope (slit lamp)

earlier: your eyelids, lashes, surrounding tissues, then the cornea, the sclera, the conjunctiva, and the inside front portion of your eyeball, especially the lens of the eye and the surrounding aqueous fluid. This examination takes about 30 seconds.

Next will be a test of your peripheral visual field. The doctor will cover one of your eyes at a time and ask you to focus the other on an object directly in front of you (usually the doctor's nose). He will then move a pen back and forth in the outer ranges of the normal visual perimeter and ask you if you see the pen moving. The test will then be repeated for the other eye. This is a *gross visual field test.* If there is a defect in your visual field, you will not see the pen when it is in the defective area, and a more detailed visual field test will have to be done. You could, of course, move your eyeball to see the pen, but that would not be a test of peripheral vision. This is why the doctor keeps a close watch to see that your gaze remains fixed on his or her nose throughout the test.

Eyedrops

Up to this point, nothing has been done to alter the way your eyes work, but now comes the part of the examination that many patients find uncomfortable—the eyedrops. Drops are a valuable and essential diagnostic tool, and it will perhaps alleviate much of the anxiety and discomfort you feel about them if you understand how they work and why they are used.

The general action of the most commonly used drops is twofold; they dilate the pupil so the interior anatomy of the eye can be examined, and they temporarily paralyze the near-focusing muscles of the eye so that an accurate refractive reading can be taken. The temporary paralysis is needed in patients under age 40 or 45 because they generally still have strong focusing ability. The findings would therefore be distorted if the eye could make its own focusing adjustments as the doctor tried to complete the examination. After age 45 or so, focusing ability is no longer a factor, so only drops that dilate the eyes will be used. Whether or not paralyzing drops are used for patients in their low- to mid-40s depends on the individual patient.

After the eyedrops are put in, you will be taken to the waiting room and will remain there briefly until they take effect; approximately 20 to 30 minutes are needed to get a full dilation with either type.

You might be relieved to know that most doctors do not

use drops that paralyze the near-focusing muscles every time they do a routine eye exam. If you are over 16 and are returning for a regular examination visit, the doctor will probably use drops that dilate only, since he or she will already have an accurate measurement of your optics and it is unlikely that they will have changed considerably. Obviously, if the examination or your complaints suggest the need for an examination with the paralyzing drops, they will have to be used. Sometimes very young children, whose focusing muscles are still very strong, and particularly young, very dark-eyed children, who have more pigment in their eyes, have a great natural resistance to the paralytic action of the most commonly used drops; stronger drops therefore have to be used. Because these eyedrops take longer to work, parents are usually given the prescription for the drops and instructions for their use. The drops can be put in at home before a second visit, when the post-drop portion of the exam will be done.

Because all these drops take some time to wear off, they sometimes cause patient discomfort. Light is irritating because the dilated pupils are unable to constrict to exclude excessive light (sunglasses will help alleviate this problem). Also, vision is blurred up close when the near-focusing muscles have been paralyzed. The effects of simple dilating drops last about three hours, while the drops that dilate and paralyze may remain in effect for as long as 24 hours. The stronger drops used for some young children can last for two days or more, depending on the type used. In all cases, the action is temporary and completely harmless.

Refraction Tests

As soon as you have the appropriate drops in your eyes and they have taken effect, the eye doctor is ready to perform a final series of tests and examination procedures. The first of these is called the *refraction,* and it is a check for corrective lenses. By now the doctor knows many things about your eyes, but only by examining your optical system with a special instrument can he or she determine whether you are nearsighted, farsighted, astigmatic, or have no optical error at all.

There are two main stages in the refraction, one objective and the other subjective. Doctors use the subjective portion to confirm the objective findings and to provide a double check and refinement. But even without your own responses to the subjective portion, an eye doctor can make a finding that is at least 95-percent accurate, close enough for all practical purposes. That is why very young children or mentally handicapped adults can still be fitted with an extremely accurate prescription. Patients who are able to cooperate on the subjective portion often feel somewhat insecure about their responses, and fear they might give the "wrong" answer and receive the wrong prescription. Such concern is unfounded because the major part of the findings comes from the objective measurement. Any response you make that contradicts these observations will be double-checked.

Two instruments are used for the objective portion. One is a *retinoscope* and the other a *phoroptor,* which contains various lenses that can be used singly or in combination to give all the possible optical corrections. The doctor will shine a light from the retinoscope into your eye and ask you to look at the light while he or she looks into your eye through the retinoscope and phoroptor, changing lenses until obtaining an almost exact measurement of your optics. In this way the doctor can determine what prescription would be required to correct your optical error, if indeed you have one. Each eye is examined separately, since the precise optics of each are usually not identical.

The subjective portion will bring this measurement as close as possible to 100-percent accuracy. This is when the doctor asks you to read the Snellen chart again while he or she holds up one of two lenses over the eye that is reading and asks you which one looks clearer. This part of the exam makes some patients nervous because the difference between the two lenses is very slight and they worry about choosing the wrong one. Again, do not be concerned about this. The eye doctor has objective findings to guide him and will not let a "wrong" answer pass without double-checking.

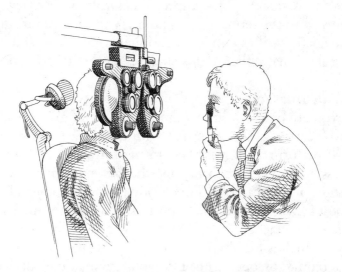

Fig. 2.6 Patient behind phoropter being examined for glasses. Doctor holds a retinoscope.

An automated refractor is used in some offices. This computer-guided instrument, which is operated by a technician, prints out the data on a strip of paper that resembles a cash register receipt. It is a somewhat less reliable method of refracting than the traditional one.

You will be returned to the biomicroscope for the next post-drop examination. Using magnification, light, and the microscopic features of the instrument, the doctor will look through your enlarged pupil all the way to the back of your eyes. Your pupil is, after all, a two-way window, so just as you can look through it out at the world, your doctor can look through it into your eye. Because your eye is filled with clear structures from front to back, the doctor's view takes him or her through the cornea, the anterior chamber, the pupil, the lens, and back to the vitreous fluid. With your now-dilated pupil, a special lens gives a clear view all the way to the retina. At this point, with the pupil dilated, the doctor will examine the periphery of the lens. If nothing abnormal is found, this check takes about 30 seconds.

Glaucoma Test

If you are over 40, have a family history of glaucoma, or show certain signs associated with the disease, the doctor will perform a *tonometry* test to measure your intraocular pressure. He will probably anesthetize your eyeballs with drops (proparacaine hydrochloride is an example) and use one of two instruments. The most commonly used is a *tonometer* attached to the biomicroscope. A special orange dye, which is highlighted under the blue light emitted by the biomicroscope, is put into your eyes. Tears will wash away the dye completely within a few minutes, so be assured that you will not leave the office with strange-looking orange eyes. The second instrument is a type of hand-held tonometer. You will sit in a tilted chair and look at the ceiling while the tonometer is applied to each of your anesthetized eyes. Each method takes less than five seconds and is completely painless.

Retina Check

The last examination procedure is performed for a closer look at the inside back of the eye. You will be asked to fix your gaze across a darkened room, and then, holding an instrument that shines a bright light through a lens system, the doctor will get close to you and look through the dilated pupil. The instrument used is called an *ophthalmoscope,* and it is like a searchlight with which the doctor can actually see your retina, including the macula, optic disc,

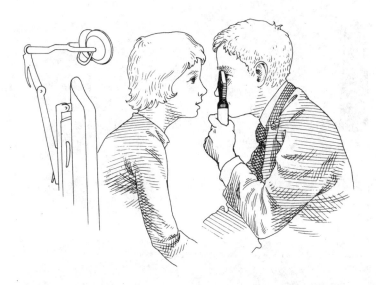

Fig. 2.7   Patient being examined with ophthalmoscope

and blood vessels of the retina. In this way, the doctor can check to see if the retina is healthy and if the circulatory system is in good condition.

The routine examination is now complete. If you wear contact lenses, they will now be checked and examined under the biomicroscope to see how well they fit and what condition they are in.

In 15 to 20 minutes (not counting the time you spent waiting for the dilating drops to take effect) the doctor has conducted as many as 20 screening tests and diagnostic examinations and has determined the following:

· the medical health of your eyes, both externally and internally

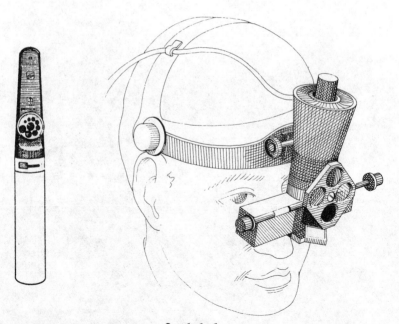

Fig. 2.8   Two types of ophthalmoscope

- your visual acuity
- your visual field
- the condition and development of your eye-muscle coordination
- whether or not you need optical correction and what your exact prescription will be if you do
- if you have cataracts
- if you might possibly have glaucoma

In short, the doctor now has a complete medical picture of your eyes. If the results of all the screening tests are normal, you have medically healthy eyes. If you have any abnormalities, further testing must be done.

In the Consultation Room

At the conclusion of the examination, the doctor will invite you into his consultation room to discuss the findings with you and go over whatever instructions and prescriptions these findings require. A responsible doctor will be more than willing to take the time to explain the findings in greater detail and to answer any pertinent questions you might have. Especially if you are the kind of patient who is comfortable only when you are confident you have been fully informed, you should by all means ask as many questions as necessary until you are sure about the doctor's findings in the examination. Your doctor should understand your need for information and should be happy to provide it.

The Optical Errors:
Nearsightedness, Farsightedness, Astigmatism, and Presbyopia

◇

MYTH: Nearsightedness and farsightedness are opposites. Nearsighted people see well up close and poorly at a distance, whereas farsighted people see well at a distance and poorly close up.

FACT: These terms refer to relative points of focus within the eye, not to the distance at which we see best. Although it is true that nearsighted people have difficulty seeing distant objects, many cannot get a clear close-up image either. On the other hand, how well a farsighted person sees—up close or at a distance—depends on the degree of the optical error *and* on how much the near-focusing muscles compensate for the farsightedness. This latter ability varies with age.

MYTH: You get more farsighted or less nearsighted as you approach middle age.

FACT: Both farsightedness and nearsightedness tend to

stabilize at about age 21. The condition people are referring to when they make the above claim is called *presbyopia,* which is a natural process of aging that affects everyone. Presbyopia is simply the loss of the ability to focus on near objects. It is not the same as farsightedness and has no effect on the ability to see distant objects clearly.

MYTH: If you do not see well at a distance, your eyes are weak.

FACT: Poor distance vision can be caused by one of several optical errors, none of which has anything to do with eye weakness or eye disease. The word *weak* implies that an eye has a muscle problem or that it is diseased or prone to disease. This is absolutely false. Optical errors do not mean that the eyes are unhealthy in any way.

Nearsightedness, farsightedness, astigmatism, and *presbyopia* are the most common eye problems, and they are the overwhelming reasons why people wear glasses or contact lenses. But there is great confusion and misunderstanding concerning these problems.

The most important point to make about these four conditions is that they are optical errors, not eye diseases. Such errors can be corrected and normal vision achieved. Eyes that are nearsighted, farsighted, astigmatic, or presbyopic are not unhealthy, nor are they more susceptible to eye disease than eyes without optical error. And by no means is blindness the ultimate outcome of any of these four conditions. The remedy for optical errors is corrective lenses— either glasses or contact lenses—which will allow perfect or near-perfect vision when they are worn. In no case can glasses or contact lenses *cure* these conditions and make it possible to see well without corrective lenses. Nothing—

including eye exercises, surgery (radial keratotomy is one external procedure), or specially designed contact lenses—can alter the internal optics of the eye.

What Is Normal Vision?

Optical errors are therefore not eye diseases but specific defects in the internal optics of the eye that prevent normal vision. *Normal vision* is a very specific term that describes the ability to see 20/20 with both eyes and to use both eyes together to deliver a visual message to the brain.

Just about everyone has heard the term 20/20 used as the ideal measurement of vision, but many do not know what it means. Most people assume it describes the two eyes in relation to each other. In fact, each eye is measured separately for *20/20 vision;* the ratio refers to the difference in acuity between the eye being measured and a theoretical normal-seeing eye. For example 20/20 vision in one eye means that eye sees at 20 feet what a normal eye can see at 20 feet. On the other hand, 20/400 vision in an eye means that you must be as close as 20 feet in order to see what a normal eye sees at 400 feet. That eye has considerably less than normal vision. A 20/15 eye can see at 20 feet what a normal eye must be within 15 feet to see, and thus is better than normal. Often the vision in both of our eyes is the same, but it is not unusual to have one eye 20/20 and the other 20/100 or whatever.

As to what the worst possible vision is, there is no limit; some people can be measured at 20/6000 or even worse.

Vision is measured both at a distance and close up. Eye doctors take the measurement for *distance vision* at 20 feet and for *near vision* at a normal reading distance, or about 14

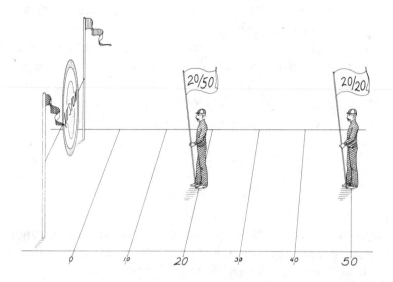

Fig. 3.1 The man with 20/20 vision can see the vision chart clearly from 50 yards away. The man with 20/50 vision must move to the 20-yard line to see it as clearly.

inches. Near vision is the vision we need for reading, sewing, eating, drawing, or any other situation in which the object viewed is within arm's reach. In practical terms, distance vision would be anything beyond that. Many people say they think of distance vision as looking at things really far away, but watching television or looking at people just across a room involves distance vision, too. *Middle distance vision,* which is neither near nor far, is not part of the ophthalmological measurement, but it does play a part in the viewing experience, particularly as one gets older. Middle-distance viewing situations include such activities as reading piano music, cooking, or playing cards. (The cards you hold require near vision; the cards across the table are beyond arm's reach but not that far away.)

Many people tend to assume that the glasses they wear to correct a distance vision problem are needed only for viewing faraway objects. But for people with optical errors, the distance for which they require correction begins at the point where they start to experience difficulty in seeing clearly.

Nearsightedness

Myopia is the technical term for nearsightedness. Although many people, including doctors, prefer to use the common name, "nearsightedness" is a bit of a misnomer for the condition. First of all, nearsightedness sounds like an advantage rather than a vision problem. Although it is true that nearsighted people see better close up than they do at a distance, they do not see better close up than people with normal vision. Very nearsighted people, for example, cannot see well whether they are at a normal reading distance or far away, and may have to hold objects very close to their eyes to be able to see them clearly without correction. Less nearsighted people may be able to see quite well at conversational distances, but have trouble seeing clearly across a room. The farther away an object is, the more blurred it appears. The more nearsighted a person is, the closer to the eyes that blur begins.

Let's review for a moment what happens when someone with normal vision looks at an object. Light rays travel from the object to the eyes. They enter the eye through the cornea, which bends the rays slightly inward so that they are no longer parallel. They then travel through the lens, which narrows them even more. The rays continue to approach each other until they converge, and are in focus when they reach the retina. The retina in turn receives the light rays and sends a message of the visual image to the brain. But the retina can send to the brain only as good an image as it receives. If the image is in sharp focus, a sharp, clear picture will be perceived. If it is not in focus, the brain will have to try to make sense out of a blurred image.

In the nearsighted eye, the light rays converge and become focused before they get to the retina. From that point, they start to diverge and go out of focus. This means that by the time light rays reach the retina, they are no longer focused. The retina sends that unfocused message to the brain, and a blurred picture is perceived. How blurred the picture is depends on how far in front of the retina the point of focus actually is. The point can be pretty close, which results in only a slight blur, or it can be quite far in front, which results in a more striking blur.

A number of different factors can cause nearsightedness. The most common is an eyeball that is longer than normal, requiring the light to travel a greater distance after it has entered the eye. But before you run to the mirror to see if your eyeball is too long, it should be explained that this refers to the distance from the front to the back of the eyeball, something you cannot see. It has nothing to do with whether your eyes look prominent or bulging. Besides, the eyeball is small enough that the tiniest variation in length is enough to make a difference. Another cause of nearsightedness can be an eye whose *refractive ability* is too great to bring an image to focus itself precisely on the retina.

Patients often ask what has caused their nearsightedness, but the underlying cause cannot be determined and cannot

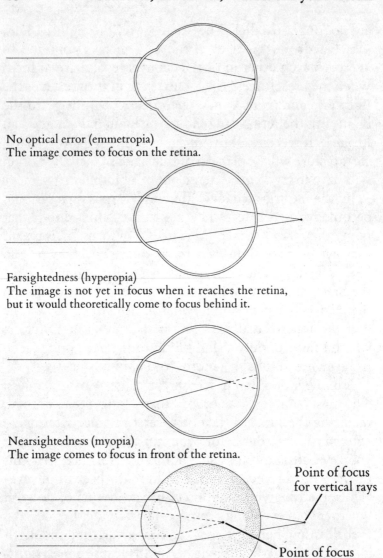

No optical error (emmetropia)
The image comes to focus on the retina.

Farsightedness (hyperopia)
The image is not yet in focus when it reaches the retina,
but it would theoretically come to focus behind it.

Nearsightedness (myopia)
The image comes to focus in front of the retina.

Point of focus
for vertical rays

Point of focus
for horizontal rays

Astigmatism
The image comes to focus at two separate points.

Fig. 3.2

be eliminated. No doctor can alter the optical system you have inherited, shorten the eyeball in any way, or prescribe eye exercises to cure this condition. All that can safely be done to compensate for this condition is to prescribe corrective lenses that help do the job the nearsighted eye cannot do for itself. There is currently a controversial operation called *radial keratotomy,* in which a physician uses a laser to scar and reshape the cornea, externally affecting the optical system (see page 103). Also, research is currently being done in which a physician uses a laser to trim part of the cornea and reshape it, theoretically reducing nearsightedness. This procedure, *photorefractive keratotomy,* may bear watching in the years ahead.

Nearsighted people can achieve slightly greater visual clarity by squinting. This is somewhat like closing down the aperture of a camera to increase depth of focus, but it certainly does not work as well as corrective lenses, and it can cause eyestrain and headaches. It is also not very attractive.

Nearsightedness usually begins to be noticeable during our growth years, which end around age 20 or 21. During this time, the statistical probability is that the degree of nearsightedness increases until the end of the period and then stabilizes. Naturally, people are not statistics, and in any individual case the degree of nearsightedness may remain the same throughout the growth years. Or the condition can even improve, although this is quite uncommon. Because of subtle refractive changes brought about by metabolic changes in the tissues of the lens or cornea, or in the fluids of the eye, nearsightedness can also get worse or better after an individual has reached adulthood. These changes, however, are usually much less marked than those that occur before adulthood. In advancing age, any cataract that develops will probably make the patient more nearsighted.

The tendency of nearsightedness to get worse during the growth years has given rise to the term *progressive myopia.* This is an unfortunate term because it suggests a disease that increases in severity. First of all, myopia is a condition, not a disease, and although it can worsen as the eyes grow, it usually stops its progression by age 21. After that point, it is unusual to get more nearsighted. Even if the nearsightedness progresses further, there is no need to fear becoming so nearsighted that you go blind. Many patients express this fear, but as long as vision is correctable to 20/20—which it is in over 99 percent of all cases of simple myopia—the only thing to worry about is the nuisance of having to wear corrective lenses.

Farsightedness

Hyperopia, or farsightedness, is another optical error. As with nearsightedness, its common name is a confusing way of referring to the condition. For one thing, the effect it has on vision is not the opposite of nearsightedness. A farsighted person does not see well at a distance and sees badly close up, whereas a nearsighted person sees better up close than at a distance. The practical effects of farsightedness are not so simple to understand as that of nearsightedness because, in addition to the degree of the error, the age of the individual is an important factor. A young farsighted person may have no problem seeing well both up close and at a distance; an older farsighted person may see equally poorly near and far.

In a farsighted eye the light rays are not yet in focus when they reach the retina. Some explanations of farsightedness are that the light rays come to focus *behind* the retina. This is not the best way to describe the condition because it suggests that the rays pass through the retina and come into focus at some point past the retina. Because the retina is opaque, light stops there, and the state of focus at that point determines the quality of the picture delivered to the brain. If light could go farther, it would focus at a certain hypothetical point, and the farther that hypothetical point lies beyond the retina, the greater the farsightedness.

But the important thing to remember is that the rays of light are *not* in focus when they arrive at the retina, and this is what causes the blurred vision of farsightedness.

It may be easier to understand and distinguish between nearsightedness and farsightedness if you think about them in the following way: The point of focus in nearsightedness is on the *near* side of the retina; the point of focus in farsightedness is on the (theoretical) *far* side of the retina. This may help avoid the confusion that comes from considering the problem as simply the nearness or farness of the object being seen.

The tricky aspect about all this is that whereas nearsighted people can do nothing to improve their vision without corrective lenses, young farsighted people can. This is what makes the chronological age of the farsighted person an important influence on what his or her vision problems are.

The near-focusing muscles, which are located inside the eye and normally used to bend the lens to bring near objects into focus, are also used by the younger farsighted eye to bring *distant* objects into focus. This is not a voluntary action that can be accomplished at will, like raising an arm or bending a leg. It happens without the individual noticing it. A person who corrects farsightedness with near-focusing muscles may have 20/20 vision and no problem seeing at a distance. But because this uses muscles intended only for focusing on near objects, eyestrain and headaches may result. The near-focusing muscles are now being used all the time, not just for near viewing as nature intended. The resultant state of constant spasm can cause secondary symptoms.

But if a farsighted person can read an eye chart as well as a person with normal vision, how will the eye doctor know a problem exists? One clue will be complaints of headaches and eyestrain, but even without such clues there is a foolproof way to uncover farsightedness, whether or not the patient is making corrections with the near-focusing muscles. The special eyedrops doctors use when they examine eyes contain a substance to paralyze the near-focusing muscles temporarily, making it possible to measure optical error without inteference from those muscles.

Besides causing headaches and eyestrain, another disadvantage in using one's near-focusing muscles to correct farsightedness is that it is a tool available only to the young. As a farsighted person gets older, the lens-bending ability of these muscles decreases until finally, by the mid-50s to 60 years of age, they will be of no use at all, either for near or far vision. The lens at this age tends to be larger, less elastic, and may soon thereafter begin to show the earliest signs of cataract formation. It is for this reason that farsighted people may not realize they have the condition until they approach middle age. This does not mean, as many people suppose, that they have suddenly developed "progressive hyperopia." Rather, they are gradually losing their innate ability to correct their farsightedness and are thus noticing long-standing vision problems for the first time.

Some degree of farsightedness is normal in growing chil-

Accommodation (focusing)

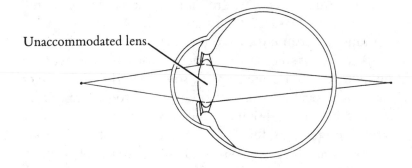

Unaccommodated lens

An image brought to focus (theoretically) behind the retina in an unaccommodated (unfocused) eye

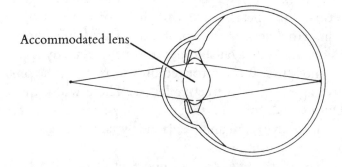

Accommodated lens

The same eye with an image brought to focus on the retina through accommodation (focusing)

Fig. 3.3 **The eye can also involuntarily use the normal process of accommodation to correct farsightedness. Viewing a distant object, the near-focusing muscles are used to bring the image forward to the retina.**

dren because the eyeball has not reached adult size and shape. Ideally, the farsightedness decreases as the eyeball grows. (And, of course, growing children usually do not need to wear glasses for the slight farsightedness normal in childhood because they can use their very strong focusing muscles to overcome the optical error.) If, however, an individual reaches age 21 with some farsightedness, he or she will probably remain that farsighted for the rest of his or her life. Farsightedness does not generally get worse after the age of 21, for, like nearsightedness, it tends to stabilize when the eyeball stops growing. Remember, however, that these are probabilities, so any one person's experience might be different.

Farsightedness can be caused by an eyeball that is slightly shorter than normal or by an eye whose light-bending ability is less than that required to deliver a focused image to the retina. Like nearsightedness, the root cause is often impossible to determine and primarily of academic interest only, since the only available and reasonable remedy is correction, not cure. If the error requires correction, the only effective approach is corrective lenses. These will provide good vision and, for younger farsighted people, relieve the symptoms of eyestrain and headache by taking the burden off the near-focusing muscles.

The lens of the eye is very important in bending light rays so that the eye is refractively normal. If the lens is removed, as in cataract surgery, the eye will be very farsighted.

Astigmatism

Astigmatism is an optical error that is caused by a variation in the shape of the cornea. Rays of light pass through the cornea on two planes—vertical and horizontal. The normal cornea is shaped like a perfect hemisphere, with the same degree of slope on each plane. This makes the rays of light come together at a single point on their way to the retina. In the astigmatic eye, one corneal plane is steeper than the other, so the rays of light do not come together at the same point. Instead, two separate images are focused at two separate points along the visual axis. One point could be on the retina and the other in front, or one could be on the retina and the other (theoretically) behind it. They could also both be in front or both behind the retina. The type of astigmatism is named for the location of the points of focus: *nearsighted astigmatism, farsighted astigmatism,* or *mixed astigmatism.*

The fact that there are two points of focus does not mean that astigmatic people see double. The effect is simply a blur, which is experienced both for distance and for near vision. The greater the distance between the two points of focus, the more astigmatic the person will be and the greater the blur he or she will perceive. Astigmatic people may also suffer from eyestrain, caused principally by squinting in an attempt to "sharpen" the image.

Astigmatism tends to develop during the growth years. It is most likely that the general degree of astigmatism you have at age 21 will remain the same for the rest of your life. It is certainly not impossible, however, for the degree of astigmatism to worsen or get better in any individual case.

Unlike farsightedness, astigmatism cannot be corrected with the near-focusing muscles, since the error is in the shape of the cornea. Often the astigmatism is insignificant and does not cause eyestrain, but if the astigmatism or discomfort from eyestrain is bad enough, corrective lenses are the only possible solution.

Presbyopia

Presbyopia is the fourth optical error, and it is the only one of the four that we are all certain to acquire at some point in our lives. Unlike the other three, which are really structural defects, presbyopia is part of the natural process of aging. And, also unlike them, presbyopia is a visual problem experienced only when looking at objects close at hand.

In simple terms, presbyopia is the loss of our ability to use the near-focusing muscles. It is what makes people need reading glasses when they reach their mid-40s. And, of course, it is the condition in the case of older farsighted people who are no longer able to correct their optical error on their own.

The near-focusing muscles bend the lens to enable us to focus on near objects. As we grow older, the lens gets more rigid and more difficult to bend. This is a process that goes on throughout life and culminates at about age 55 to 60, at which time all lens-bending ability is lost. This is a predictable phenomenon—so predictable, in fact, that your eye doctor can determine your age with great accuracy simply by taking into account your optical error (if any) and then observing how close up you can focus. So be warned: Even if you can fool your friends, you can't hide your age from your eye doctor.

Young children are able to focus on an object held very close to their eyes. The point at which it is possible to focus gradually recedes as we grow older, but it presents no practical problem until it gets beyond comfortable reading range. This happens in the mid-40s and is the time when people start joking that their arms are not long enough to hold a book.

Presbyopia is not the same thing as farsightedness. Something entirely different is going on inside the eye, and blurred vision is present only when the eye views nearby objects. Distance vision is not affected by presbyopia at all. In fact, one can be presbyopic and farsighted (or nearsighted or astigmatic) at the same time. If you have an optical error as a young adult, you will still have it in addition to the symptoms of presbyopia beginning in your mid-40s.

The correction for presbyopia is reading glasses. These need to be worn for any kind of close-viewing situation. A person who has no other optical error will need reading glasses only. A person who wears glasses to correct another optical error may need to wear bifocals or own two separate pairs of glasses, one for seeing at a distance and one for near objects.

Between the ages of 40 and 60, when the focusing ability is noticeably declining, frequent changes of a prescription are required. By the mid-50s to 65 years of age, all focusing ability is lost and your presbyopia cannot get worse.

It should now be clear that the four eye problems under discussion are imperfections of the optical system, not diseases. The treatments are not cures but corrective measures. It is important to emphasize this point once more by saying that eyes with optical defects are not diseased eyes. There is no reason to fear blindness as the end result of an optical error. The important thing to remember is that an eye doctor can correct optical errors. This will mean wearing glasses or contact lenses to see well, but even dependence on them cannot be considered any more than a nuisance.

Correcting Optical Errors:
Eyeglasses and Contact Lenses

◇

MYTH: Wearing glasses will weaken your eyes or, conversely, wearing glasses will strengthen them.

FACT: These contradictory notions are equally false. Glasses correct optical errors when they are worn, but they have no effect—good or bad—on the optical system within the eye and therefore do not make the eyes weaker or stronger.

The idea that glasses do the work instead of your eyes is probably at the root of each of these myths. Some people assume that "vacationing" eyes are getting stronger because they do not have to work so hard, whereas others believe that the eyes get weaker from lack of visual exercise. Both ideas are absurd. When you wear glasses your eyes are working just as hard as they do when you are not wearing glasses. The only difference is that you see better when glasses do what your eyes cannot do alone.

MYTH: If you have 20/20 vision, it definitely means you do not need glasses.

FACT: Oddly enough, this is not true. For example, young people who are very farsighted can use their strong near-focusing muscles to see clearly at the distance and thus correct their farsightedness. A simple test of their vision will yield a reading of 20/20, but the constant use of these muscles for other than their intended function can cause eye fatigue, eyestrain, and headaches, especially while reading. Glasses will alleviate the symptoms and allow 20/20 vision without taxing those muscles.

MYTH: Tinted glasses are bad for your eyes and should not be worn indoors.

FACT: Slightly or heavily tinted glasses can be worn for their cosmetic effect or to shield the eyes from glare or bright sunlight, but they are of no proven medical benefit or disadvantage. You can even wear sunglasses indoors where the light intensity is low without endangering your sight in any way. Doing so is not recommended, however, since it makes seeing more difficult, but that is simply because the tinted lenses reduce the amount of light by which you see, not because they endanger your eyes. Common sense dictates not using tinted lenses for night driving.

MYTH: Contact lenses are not really safe, and lots of people have trouble wearing them.

FACT: Contact lenses are just about as safe as eyeglasses, and the overwhelming majority of people who try them can wear them with no difficulty at all. As long as the contacts are fitted by or under the direction of an ophthalmologist, are hygienically cared for and inserted and removed according to your doctor's instructions, and are checked regularly by your eye doctor, there is no reason why you cannot wear them safely and comfortably.

MYTH: Contact lenses cure astigmatism.
FACT: Astigmatism cannot be cured. However, because astigmatism is caused by an irregularity in the surface of the cornea, rigid contact lenses provide an intrinsic correction for the condition. If rigid contacts are worn, the perfect curve of the contact lens replaces the astigmatic cornea as the light-bending surface.

Eyeglasses

Eyeglasses have been around for at least a thousand years. Indeed, there is evidence that the ancient Egyptians and Assyrians used some sort of magnifying lenses to improve their vision. No single individual can be identified as the inventor of eyeglasses. By the tenth century glasses turned up simultaneously in such distant and unrelated places as Europe and China. When Marco Polo made his journey to the East, he observed that the Chinese used specially ground lenses to read fine print and unground colored crystals to protect their eyes from the sun's glare.

In Europe during the Middle Ages, monks were just about the only beneficiaries of improved sight through glasses. As a literate elite in an age of mass illiteracy, these men were among the few who needed to have perfect vision. This does not mean that kings and peasants, farmers and Crusaders, courtiers and serving maids did not have eye problems. It simply means that their visual needs were not great enough to justify the use of glasses—their vision problems were just not enough of a nuisance to interfere with the way they spent their time. And although the ways we spend our time today are quite different, the same principle still applies.

Eyeglasses will help correct any of the four optical errors discussed in the last chapter and will relieve secondary symptoms of these errors. But they do this when, and only when, they are worn. Whether or not a person wears glasses depends not only on how great that person's optical error is but also on the extent of the demand the person puts on the eyes in various viewing situations and how important it is to see better. The monk who spent hours reading the Bible and copying manuscripts had to have very good vision. Because he spent so much time reading, vision problems caused serious disruptions of his daily life, and if the optical error were of the type that causes eyestrain and headaches, the symptoms would be severe. On the other hand, a warrior or tiller of the soil could accomplish his daily tasks without perfectly acute vision; because he did not demand as much from his eyes, any secondary symptoms would seem less severe.

Today, with wider literacy and a greater range of tasks that require close vision, even people who are not scholars choose to wear glasses if they need help in achieving good vision. But in many marginal cases the decision remains a matter of choice. The four factors that go into making that choice are: How bad is the optical error? Are you bothered by secondary symptoms? How much demand do your work and your life-style put on your eyes? How well do you need to see to feel comfortable in your environment? A misunderstanding of any of these factors, or about their relation to each other, can be a source of great confusion.

Glasses are essentially a prosthetic device, like false teeth, which are not essential to your health but nice to have if you want to be able to chew certain foods. Or like elevator shoes for short people. There is nothing unhealthy about being short, but elevator shoes will make an individual who is bothered by being short look taller. As soon as you have removed the shoes, of course, the height you gained is lost until you put the shoes on again.

If you have an optical error, even a great one, but choose not to wear glasses, you will not be endangering the health of your eyes. The only exceptions to this rule are young children with eye problems that, left untreated, could result in a permanent inability to develop normal sight. Although the choice is a free one for the rest of us, most people will opt for the improved vision and greater comfort that wearing glasses can provide.

What Types of Glasses Are There?

Eyeglasses are specially ground lenses that are custom-made to the optics of the individual eye. Their function is always to deliver a focused image to the retina. Eyeglass lenses are worn outside the eye and form a surface through which light passes on its way from the object to the eye. The optical center of the lens is a tiny point positioned directly in front of the pupil. When light passes through the optical center, it is bent in a way that compensates for the eye's inability to bend the light correctly.

The most commonly prescribed type of eyeglass is called the *single-vision lens.* Its name does not mean it is for seeing at one distance only; it can be a reading glass or a distance glass, or it can be worn for seeing both close up and at a distance. Single vision simply means that there is only one

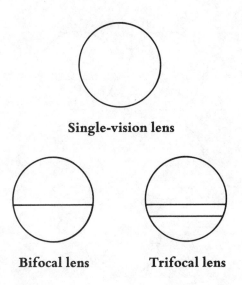

Single-vision lens

Bifocal lens   **Trifocal lens**

Fig. 4.1   Three basic lens types

set of optical corrections in the lens. This distinguishes it from the second most common type, the *bifocal*.

Bifocals contain two sets of optical corrections, one in the upper portion of the lens and the other in the lower portion. The most common application for bifocals is for people who are presbyopic and have another optical error that needs correcting for good vision at the distance. The top portion is for viewing distant objects and contains the correction for the distance optical error only (nearsightedness, farsightedness, or astigmatism). The bottom portion is for reading; it contains a combination of the presbyopic correction and the correction for the other optical error, the one represented in the upper portion.

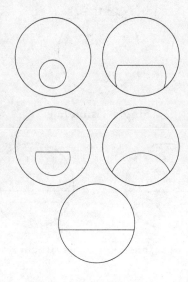

Fig. 4.2   Some bifocal lens shapes

Although it usually takes a while to get accustomed to bifocals, most people are able to use them comfortably, because we tend to look down when we read and straight ahead when we look at objects farther away. By keeping the eyeglass centered in front of our eyes and just moving each eyeball, we are able to look through the proper portion of the lens. The most frequent adjustment problem bifocal wearers have occurs when they walk up or down stairs. The difficulty here is that the distance between eyes and feet is great enough to require distance correction, but we must look down (or into the near-vision part of the lens) to see where we are stepping. It is advisable for bifocal patients to drop their chins all the way down when using stairs or stepping off curbs, so they will be looking through the top of their bifocals. Developing this habit usually solves the problem.

Bifocals are never absolutely necessary, but they are convenient since they make it unnecessary to change glasses every time you want to change from near to distance vision and back. However, some people think bifocals will give away their age, so they prefer to put up with the inconveniences of using two pairs of glasses. Such inconvenience can be considerable for people whose daily activities require that they see well at both distances in close succession.

There are numerous designs available in bifocal correction. Many years ago most bifocals allocated only a small rounded portion near the bottom for near-vision correction. There has been a tendency in recent decades to devote a greater part of the total glass area to near-vision correction. In most bifocal glasses, whatever the division between distant- and near-vision areas, the line separating the two areas is visible on the glass. However, bifocals with no obvious division between the two areas are also available. In these, the demarcation line is ground smooth, so the wearer sees a blurred strip rather than a sharp line of demarcation. Thus, the fact that the glasses are bifocals is not evident to the outside world.

Another kind of bifocal can be worn by people who are presbyopic but who have no other optical error. The bottom portion contains the correction for their presbyopia, while the top is plain glass with no correction at all. To read, the wearer looks down and through the presbyopic correction; for distance viewing the wearer looks up and through unground glass. Half glasses are another version of the same principle. In this case, the wearer looks through air when he or she looks up. The advantage of either of these types is that the wearer does not have to don glasses for reading and remove them to see clearly in the distance. The disadvantage of half glasses is that they encourage a chin-down posture of the head that many associate with advancing age.

Trifocals give the wearer correction at three rather than two viewing distances, adding a middle-distance correction between the distant and close viewing areas. Although tri-focals work well once the wearer becomes accustomed to them, the adjustment is difficult for many people. Most eye doctors are reluctant to prescribe them unless a special occu-pational need exists.

Another variation on bifocal and trifocal lenses is one that has a gradually changing focal length, top to bottom. It corrects for far viewing at the top of the glass, gradually becoming a correction for the so-called middle-distance viewing in the mid-height area of the lens, until a correc-tion for near vision is provided at the bottom. This design has several advantages. Like the smooth-line bifocal, it dis-plays no telltale bifocal line to others. As well, the wearer does not have a blurred area across his vision as he or she would with a smooth-line bifocal. Those who need trifo-cals may find this kind of correction, which provides even more than three corrections, useful. Unfortunately, many patients, particularly those with little or no distance optical error, have enormous difficulty getting used to this kind of corrective lens.

If bifocals are needed, the eye doctor has to decide which type to prescribe in close consultation with the patient. Most patients will likely find that a larger close-viewing area clearly separated from the distance portion is the easiest bifocal to adjust to; it is also the most practical for use in most lines of work. Those patients reluctant to display to the world that they have reached the age where bifocals have become necessary may prefer the smooth-line design, but the doctor should caution that the blur may take some getting used to. Trifocals and lenses with gradually changing focal lengths are usually reserved for special situations that call rather specifically for them.

Special Needs, Special Solutions

A number of special vocational and avocational needs might be well served by unconventional optical solutions. The best way to approach these is through collaboration between patient and eye doctor.

For example, special glasses may be needed for computer users. The computer monitor usually lies at a middle distance. A number of possible solutions exist. One is single-vision lenses, prescribed for the distance from eye to computer screen, to be used for viewing at that distance only. A second is a bifocal with the top portion ground for the middle (eye-to-screen) distance, the bottom for near-vision work that needs to be referred to at the same time. In both of these cases no optical correction is provided for true distance vision, so the glasses would not be worn away from the workstation. A variation of the trifocal with a much wider middle-viewing area for the computer is another possibility, but this arrangement generally does not work very well because it leaves only a very small area at the top for the distance segment.

To solve this problem, an eye doctor will ask the patient to measure the exact distance from his or her eyes to the computer screen, and between the eyes and other key working distances. The patient's most important goals in terms of visual acuity are then discussed. The pros and cons of the various options should be outlined clearly before a treatment decision is reached.

A pianist or other musician who reads music on a stand middle-distant from his or her eyes also has special needs. In this case, however, single-vision lenses made for the middle distance are the best solution because that is where attention is focused. A musician who also needs to see a conductor might require bifocals with the bottom portion for middle distance and the top for the distance.

Dentists often require special bifocals for presbyopia and another optical error. Typically, a dentist leans down over a patient while looking through the top half of his or her glasses. Near vision is required to see the patient's mouth. The solution for far vision could be a bifocal with the top 33 to 40 percent of the lens for near vision and the remainder for distance vision. When the dentist lifts his or her chin slightly or looks straight ahead, the eyes will look through the lower 60 to 67 percent of the lens, allowing clear vision in the distance.

Who Needs Glasses?

If you fulfill most or all of the following interrelated conditions, you need glasses: (1) You have an optical error, (2) you find the less-than-perfect vision enough of an annoyance to want to improve it, (3) you put demands on the eyes that make the optical error a hindrance to how well you need to see, (4) this demand causes secondary symptoms of headache and eyestrain. Optical error alone, regardless of how small or great, does not mean you have to wear glasses.

How Lenses Correct Optical Errors

Each optical error is corrected with a specially shaped lens, and in each case the result is a focused image on the retina. The lens that corrects nearsightedness is a *concave lens*.

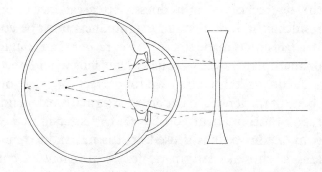

A concave lens pushes the focused rays of light backward to the retina to correct nearsightedness.

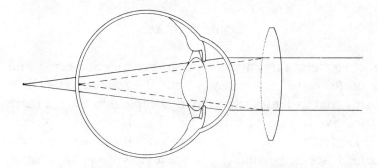

A convex lens pulls the focused rays of light forward to the retina to correct farsightedness.

Fig. 4.3

The concave shape pushes back the focused rays of light farther than the eye can do itself. This works no matter what the cause of the nearsightedness.

A *convex lens* is used to correct farsightedness. The effect here is to bring the rays of light into focus sooner than they normally would be so that a focused image is delivered to the retina. And again, the degree of convexity depends on the degree of farsightedness. After cataract surgery the resulting high degree of farsightedness must be corrected. If a decision is made to use glasses rather than contact lenses or an implant, a very strong convex lens would be required.

A convex lens is also used for correcting presbyopia. The shape of the lens used to correct astigmatism depends on the type of astigmatism you have. If it is farsighted astigmatism, a convex lens is used; if it is nearsighted, a concave lens is chosen. Astigmatic lenses also have a correction ground into them that offsets the error in slope of the cornea on whichever plane it occurs. This correction collapses the two images into one.

Contact Lenses

Contact lenses are another option open to most people who require visual correction. About 25 million Americans wear contact lenses today. Many people find them a more attractive solution to their visual problems than glasses. However, quite a few people wonder if contact lenses are safe. It seems beyond dispute that they do provide three important advantages over glasses: a more natural and attractive appearance; a fuller, unobstructed field of view; and in most cases a better correction of optical error. But the safety question still arises, probably because everyone has heard at least one contact lens disaster story and has seen at least one person on a dance floor or athletic field in panic over a lost or displaced contact lens. What is not so easy to realize is that each of us deals daily with some of the millions of people who are safely, comfortably, and uneventfully enjoying the visual benefits of this technological marvel. They are wearing contacts without our being aware that they are.

But still there are some caveats to consider. Contact lenses are completely safe *if* three cardinal rules are followed: (1) The lenses are fitted by or under the supervision of a medical contact lens specialist, (2) hygienic insertion and removal procedures are followed to the letter, and (3) both eyes and lenses are checked periodically by a medical eye doctor. These rules are easy enough to follow, so there is no reason why a person who wants contact lenses, and whose optical error lends itself to correction with them, cannot safely wear contact lenses.

Types

So-called hard contact lenses, made of light plastic, became widely popular in the 1950s. They are economical, easy to care for, last a long time, and generally provide excellent visual acuity. They do, however, require a period of adjustment for full-time wear. They occasionally move out of their position in front of the pupil and even pop out of the eye. And when a foreign body lodges under a lens, it is quite uncomfortable.

About 20 years ago soft contact lenses were introduced. For those who can wear them, they have many advantages over hard lenses: They are almost immediately comfortable, requiring virtually no adjustment period. They can be worn as desired, even if you vary the schedule from a few hours one day to all day or not at all the next, for example. They rarely permit foreign bodies to get lodged under their surface and irritate the eye, and virtually never become loosened from the eye. There are also disadvantages, however: They require far more extensive cleaning and maintenance procedures than hard lenses. They tend to wear out more rapidly, or even tear. And because of higher maintenance costs and the necessity of replacing them more frequently, they are definitely costlier. In addition, the optical correction they offer is often not as satisfactory as that of hard lenses, and for certain optical errors (most notably high degrees of astigmatism) they are not suitable at all.

About 15 years ago what are now referred to as gas-permeable rigid lenses came into ever greater use. There are now several different types with characteristic differences, depending on the material they are made of. In general, however, these rigid lenses are harder than soft lenses, but are not as hard as the original hard lenses. They do not flex as the gelatin-like plastic of soft lenses does, and they are lighter in weight than hard lenses.

This new generation of contact lenses offers improvements over both soft and hard lenses. They require less cleaning and maintenance than soft lenses but are more comfortable to wear than hard lenses because they allow more oxygen to reach the cornea. Although adequate oxygen reaches the cornea even with hard lenses, all else being equal, the more oxygen the cornea can get, the more comfortable the lens will be. Some adjustment is needed before they can be worn comfortably full-time, but the break-in period is much shorter than with hard lenses. Optically, they are superior to soft lenses yet generally the equal of hard lenses. They tend to last longer than soft lenses, and

this, along with generally less costly cleaning requirements, makes them somewhat more economical.

In the 1950s and 1960s, all contact lenses fitted in the
United States were hard lenses. Starting in the early 1970s
soft contact lenses increasingly took over the market until
they represented at their height about 80 percent of contact
lens sales. Gas-permeable rigid lenses have steadily
increased their market share since the mid-1970s and today
represent close to half of all contact lenses fitted in the
United States. The trend is definitely toward gas-
permeables, and they will likely be the predominant lens
prescribed in the future. New plastics continue to be developed for these lenses, allowing for an ever lighter and more
oxygen-permeable lens. Two that are currently in development contain fluorine, which increases stability,
durability, and oxygen permeability. Lenses made with
fluorosilicone are rigid, whereas those made with fluoro-
polymer are flexible.

How Contact Lenses Work

Contact lenses float on a layer of tears in front of the cornea
and are held in place by the surface tension of the fluid.
Since the lenses do not rest directly on the corneal tissue,
they do not interfere with its supply of oxygen. Each time
the eye blinks, tears wash under the contact, bringing a new
supply of oxygen to the cornea. The tissues of the cornea
are strong enough not to be injured by a minute, feather-
light lens floating on it, and should the lens slide off the
cornea, the sclera and conjunctiva are resistant to damage
and abrasion from the lens. In addition, the conjunctiva
closes off the back of the eye, so there is no danger that the

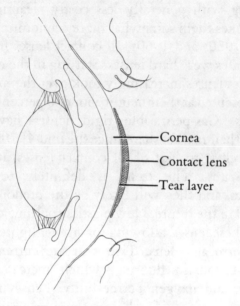

Cornea

Contact lens

Tear layer

Fig. 4.4   Contact lens in position

lens will get lost in the eye and migrate back inside the head.

All contact lenses, regardless of what they are called and how they are advertised, operate on this principle. Do not be fooled by a particular manufacturer's claims of superiority because their lens is "contactless," "free-floating," or whatever. These are simply fancy ways of saying that the lens makes no contact with the eyeball tissue or that it floats on the tear layer, or that it allows oxygen to reach the cornea—all of which are true, but certainly not features unique to any particular brand of lens. The "contact" in all contact lenses is with the tear layer and *not* with the cornea, and all lenses permit oxygen exchange through your natural tear fluid. The only significant difference in contacts is whether they are hard, rigid gas-permeable, or soft, since the plastics from which each type is made, the fitting techniques, and the wearing procedures all differ.

Hard contact lenses, which from the beginning have been made of only one type of plastic, are impervious to oxygen. That is, the corneal tissue does not receive oxygen from the air through the plastic, although it does get oxygen from tears. If a hard lens is well fitted and the wearer

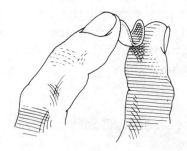

Soft contact lenses are flexible.

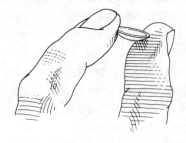

Hard contact lenses are rigid, as are the great majority of gas-permeable lenses.

Fig. 4.5

has a good blink reflex and adequate tear production, the oxygen supply to the cornea will be sufficient to maintain eye health.

Soft contact lenses, some of which are as much as 80 percent water, permit oxygen to pass through the lens to the cornea beneath it. The result may be greater wearing comfort for a longer period of time. As of this writing, there are over 50 different brands of soft contact lenses on the market. They vary in size, shape, mode of manufacture, and percentage of water content, as well as type of plastic.

Rigid gas-permeable lenses, as their name suggests, also permit oxygen to pass through the lens to the cornea. There are several types, varying in size and, depending on the type of plastic from which they are made, in degree of rigidity and gas permeability.

Glasses Versus Contact Lenses

It is popularly but incorrectly believed that the choice of contact lenses over glasses is simply a matter of vanity and, therefore, is a costly indulgence.

Contact lenses provide better optical correction than glasses in several ways. First of all, they fit in a more natural way, resting directly on the tear layer to create a uniform optical system rather like the natural tear-layer/cornea/lens system we are all born with. With glasses, on the other hand, there is a kind of triple optical system: lens, air, and the optics of the eye itself. In nearsighted individuals, who are the most typical wearers of contact lenses, the triple system of glasses makes objects look smaller—considerably so if the person is very myopic—and this can have an effect on vision. An extremely nearsighted person's vision can be corrected to very nearly 20/20 with contact lenses, but objects viewed by that same person through glasses will be made so small that 20/20 vision may not be possible. In practical terms, small equals distant, since the farther away an object is, the smaller it looks and the harder it is to see. Even if it is glasses that make the object look smaller rather than the object's distance from the eye, the effect is the same. Contact lenses, on the other hand, do not alter the size of objects at all.

Another optical advantage of contacts is that they allow normal peripheral vision, whereas the frames of glasses can obstruct vision on the side. Furthermore, people who wear glasses must move their heads when viewing objects that are not straight ahead to ensure that they are looking through the optical center of their glasses. If they rotate their eyes only, they will be looking through an area toward the edge of the glass and will get a prismatic distortion. Contact lens wearers can rotate their eyes and see clearly up, down, and on all sides. The central optical zone of contact lenses is not only proportionately much larger than that of glasses, but it is also always in front of the pupil, no matter how the eye moves. The optical benefits of contact lenses increase as the optical error increases. Hence the benefit over glasses in a person after cataract surgery is great, because there tends to be a high degree of farsightedness after the operation.

Another advantage of contact lenses is in the correction of astigmatism. By creating a perfect front surface of the eye—in effect acting as a substitute for the irregularly shaped cornea—rigid contacts automatically correct astigmatism, whereas glasses must have an astigmatic correction as part of the prescription. One of the more frequent reasons for prescription changes in glasses is not change in nearsightedness or farsightedness but a change in astigmatism. The need for change, therefore, is reduced when rigid contact lenses are worn, because a change in astigmatism does not require a new prescription. Most types of soft lenses do not confer this advantage.

In spite of these real optical advantages, for many people the main motivation for wearing contact lenses is still cosmetic. It is a fact that people look better and more natural without glasses on their faces, no matter how fashionable and attractive the eyeglass frames may be. But there is a further cosmetic advantage that many people may be unaware of: The alteration of image size works on both sides of a pair of glasses, so the eyes of the wearer, when viewed through their glasses by another person, also look different. This alteration is, in fact, much greater than the one the wearer perceives. A nearsighted person's eyes will appear quite a bit smaller than they really are, and a farsighted person's eyes will appear larger. This is not a problem with contact lenses. No image size variation is apparent from either vantage point, so the contact lens wearer's eyes look normal to the outside world just as the outside world looks normal to the wearer.

Enthusiasm on the part of wearers is always a major factor in a successful contact lens fit. People with a low tolerance for discomfort and high impatience with things that take extra time out of their day are poor contact lens candidates. People who really want contact lenses with today's latest technology can virtually always be successfully fitted and are always an eye doctor's happiest and most grateful patients.

Much is made of the discomfort and inconvenience associated with contact lenses, but there is also some appreciable inconvenience involved in wearing glasses, even though people seem more willing to accept this as a necessary evil. The pressure of eyeglasses on the ridge of the nose, the tops of the ears, and the temples often causes red marks, skin irritation, and headaches. Glasses fog up when the wearer moves between locations with markedly different temperatures. Glasses can get wet and misty, just as a car windshield does, but they rarely come equipped with windshield wipers. Contact lenses never fog up when the temperature shifts, and eyelids serve to wipe the lenses with every blink. It is true that contact lenses must be cleaned before insertion and upon removal, but most eyeglass wearers find they must wipe their glasses several times a day to keep them clean. Contact lenses are, in the final analysis, less of a nuisance than glasses.

The Use of Contact Lenses

In addition to their optical and cosmetic advantages, we can list a number of optical and medical conditions for which contact lenses are either the preferred or the only solution.

Nonmedical Uses

The most common nonmedical use is for nearsightedness, largely because this condition usually requires full-time correction. Because contact lenses (and particularly rigid lenses) are intended for regular, full-time wear, they are ideally suited for nearsighted people. Farsighted people can also wear contact lenses if their farsightedness requires full-time correction, but contacts are generally not suitable for people who need correction only for reading.

If astigmatism, with or without myopia or hyperopia,

requires full-time correction, then contacts are a good solution.

Conventional rigid contact lenses, hard or gas-permeable, automatically correct astigmatism. *Toric lenses,* which may be soft or rigid, are intended for use with moderate to severe astigmatism. Designed to remain stable on the eye without turning, toric lenses have a cylinder correction on the front surface. A more complex variation of this is the *bitoric lens,* usually reserved for severe astigmatism. Its inner surface is carved to fit the wearer's corneal surface, increasing the stability of the lens.

Fitting toric lenses is difficult and expensive, and only an estimated 50 percent of those who try them obtain a successful fit. They rarely offer advantages over conventional rigid lenses that would justify their greater expense and fitting problems.

Patients in the bifocal age group represent a particular correction problem that is solvable with contacts in one of three ways. The least desirable is bifocal contact lenses, which provide optical correction for near and far vision within the same lens.

Bifocal contacts, which may be soft or rigid, are of two main types: simultaneous-vision and alternating-vision. A simultaneous-vision contact lens resembles a target, with the bullseye for distance vision and the outer portion for near vision. The brain selects the incoming images it will recognize. The alternating-vision lens moves on the eye as the wearer looks up or down. The downward gaze is through the near or reading segment of the lens, the upward gaze through the distance segment. Alternating-vision lenses provide good vision but are difficult to fit; simultaneous-vision lenses are easier to fit, but the vision they provide is generally not as acute. With the state of the art where it currently is, neither of these lenses works terribly well and the rate of satisfied wearers is relatively low.

The second solution is to fit an eye patient with corrective lenses (rigid or soft) for distance vision in addition to reading glasses (which can be worn over the lenses for near vision). The convenience factor is somewhat reduced here, however, since glasses are needed in addition to contacts.

A third solution is to fit one eye with a contact lens to correct for distance and the other eye with a contact lens to correct for near vision. This is called the *monovision system*. Bizarre as it may sound, this setup is remarkably successful and eliminates the need for any glasses whatsoever. The reason such a method works is that it allows one eye to see well at the distance but not sharply close up, while the other eye sees well near but not sharply in the distance. Both eyes receive the image, but the one that gets the better image at any given moment tends to dominate, and the brain accepts the clearer message of the two. The wearer is not aware of the blurred image, and unless one eye is covered, the wearer will see perfectly well at all times.

This is a particularly good solution if it is chosen early in a person's bifocal years, when there is only a slight variation between the correction for near and far vision. As the variation increases, the doctor can make gradual prescription changes, which are not difficult to adjust to.

Another special nonmedical use for contacts occurs when there is an appreciable difference between the optical errors of each eye. This is difficult to correct with glasses since there is an intolerable discrepancy in the size of images seen with each eye. When contacts are used, the problem is eliminated, since both eyes can be corrected without affecting the size of images seen.

Cosmetic Uses

Purely cosmetic contact lenses are used to change eye color. They cover almost the entire cornea in order to obliterate the iris. These hard or soft lenses are opaquely colored to resemble the iris with a clear central pupil through which you see.

The quality of opaquely tinted lenses varies, along with the price, which is generally higher than standard lenses. Inexpensive cosmetic lenses are quite artificial-looking, but as the cost increases, the lenses tend to approximate the human iris more closely. There are a few medical-cosmetic applications for these lenses, such as covering a disfigured cornea that has become scarred or opaque. In such cases, the lens is made to match the other eye. Other than that, people in the performing arts who might in certain circumstances require a specific eye color other than their own are among the few for whom these lenses make sense.

Translucent tints are of value primarily for reducing glare and making the lenses more visible when they are out of the eye. Slightly darker though still translucent tints are marketed as a way to "enhance" natural eye color. As such, they work best for light-colored eyes, such as gray, green, blue, or light brown.

Medical/Optical Uses

There are several medical and optical conditions for which an eye doctor may prescribe contact lenses as treatment or correction. The most common of these is after cataract surgery, when a lens implant has not been done. Because removal of the cataractous lens will create extreme farsightedness, the image size variation caused by glasses can be very disorienting, impossibly so if only one eye has been operated on. Most people find adjustment to contact lenses easier than relearning spatial relations, and hard or soft lenses provide excellent vision without making the eyes look huge and bulging, which the very thick glasses needed after cataract surgery would do.

A medical indication for hard lenses is *keratoconus,* a disease characterized by the thinning and forward bulging of the cornea. If left untreated, the disease may progress and result in a tear of the corneal tissue that will produce scarring of the cornea, leaving the eye with decreased useful vision. A rigid contact lens pressing on the front of the cornea tends to retard the disease and permit far better vision than would be possible with glasses. The lens functions both as an optical correction (because high astigmatism is caused by the bulging cornea) and as a sort of truss to control the bulge.

Soft contact lenses are sometimes used as bandages for certain painful conditions of the cornea. They relieve the pain caused by exposure to the air and protect the diseased cornea from irritation when the eyelid opens and closes over it. This is a purely medical indication and is used only for severe, chronic disease; a doctor will not use a soft lens bandage for a minor corneal burn or abrasion, for example. No optical correction need be included in the bandage lens, although it can be added if necessary.

Contact Lens Types: Soft Versus Gas-Permeable

Although a new lens wearer should virtually never start out with hard contact lenses, if he or she has been wearing hard lenses for years, is comfortable with them, and has a healthy cornea, there is absolutely no reason to change to a new type just because newer types are available.

Today the main decision in selecting contact lenses is choosing between soft and rigid gas-permeable lenses. The appropriate choice depends largely on the wearer's disposition: how highly one's immediate comfort is valued, how often the lenses will be worn, and how diligently they will be cared for. Let us look at how the two types compare.

Comfort

The immediate comfort of soft lenses is their major advantage over rigid ones. Soft lenses require hardly any break-in time, whereas rigid lenses may take a week for adjustment. The quick adaptation to soft lenses makes them an ideal choice for people who wear contacts only occasionally.

A soft lens begins to dry out soon after it is put in, however. That can change the fit of the lens, which may cause irritation and affect vision. So wearers must commonly use eyedrops in order to keep the lens moist. A rigid lens contains virtually no water and so will not dry out.

Perhaps more important, a soft lens almost inevitably accumulates deposits and becomes less comfortable over time. A rigid lens is easier to keep clean and tends to be more comfortable than a soft lens in the long run.

Lens Care

A soft lens soaks up more than just water. Its wet, gummy surface attracts tear proteins and mucus as well as microorganisms. Unless the lens is kept scrupulously clean, deposits can build up and irritate the eye; and the microorganisms can cause corneal infections.

To keep deposits and microbes in check, soft-lens wearers must put their contacts through a costly and often complex cleaning and disinfection regimen. The hard surfaces of rigid lenses are easier to clean, however, and deposits and microorganisms do not adhere to them as readily. As a result, caring for rigid lenses is generally simpler and cheaper.

Durability

Surface deposits have shortened the life of many a soft lens. If deposits do not do them in, a scratch from a fingernail might—often while cleaning the lens. The average lifespan of a soft lens is only about nine to 12 months. Although rigid gas-permeable lenses are softer and more easily damaged than hard lenses, they can still be expected to last at least twice as long as soft lenses.

Protection from Irritants

Soft lenses offer an advantage for those who must often contend with dust and soot. The lens is larger than the cornea and fits on it snugly, preventing airborne particles from slipping under the lens and irritating the cornea. Rigid lenses are not as large as soft lenses, do not cling as snugly, and consequently provide less protection against particles of grit. The snug fit of the soft lens also makes it less likely to fall off, a plus for certain athletic activities.

Safety

Studies suggest that rigid lenses cause fewer complications than soft lenses, probably because they are easier to keep clean and less likely to cause eye infections.

When deciding which types of contact lens to get, weigh these considerations with your eye doctor. His or her knowledge of your optical error and medical eye health, combined with your own notions of your visual needs, personal habits, and temperament, will lead to the best possible choice.

Newer Lens Types

Extended-wear lenses are contacts that have been approved by the U.S. Food and Drug Administration (FDA) for 24-hour wear. You can wear them while sleeping and generally need to remove them for cleaning only once a week, or in some cases as infrequently as once a month. Most of them are soft lenses, but a few rigid, gas-permeable types have been approved for extended wear as well.

Disposable lenses are soft contacts that can be worn up to one full week, then discarded and replaced by identical new ones.

Because they eliminate the nuisance of daily cleaning, extended-wear lenses had a popular run several years ago. They were first approved by the FDA in 1981, and probably represented as much as a quarter of soft-lens sales in the mid-eighties. Increasing reports of serious infections and other problems, however, have reduced their popularity. It has become apparent that the longer the interval of wear between overnight "breathers" (leaving the lenses out overnight), the greater the risk of infection. A normal blink reflex is important to healthy, comfortable contact lens wear. We do not blink when we sleep, and so mucus and naturally occurring proteins tend to accumulate on the lens overnight, increasing the likelihood of discomfort and infections.

Today most ophthalmologists prefer to fit daily-wear soft lenses. Nonetheless, extended-wear lenses can be very useful for people with certain disabilities and can also be very useful as a temporary measure on outdoor or overnight trips, or in other special travel situations.

In general, disposable lenses are probably preferable to longer-lived extended-wear lenses because at least a new sterile lens is used weekly. If extended-wear lenses are used, more frequent ophthalmological follow-up is necessary, particularly in the first few months before the doctor has had an opportunity to observe the pattern for that patient.

Where to Get Your Contact Lenses

The prescription of contact lenses requires very precise measurements with special instruments and an examination of the health of the eyes. This should be a medical procedure, best performed by a trained *ophthalmologist.*

Fitting the increasingly popular gas-permeable lenses is far more complicated than fitting soft lenses. Soft lenses are almost never custom-made because the pliable material of which they are made conforms to nearly every eye contour. Most eye doctors carry an inventory of soft lenses, so the wearer can usually take home lenses with the specific optics needed on the very same day. Gas-permeable lenses, on the other hand, are almost always custom-made because the contours of the rigid lens must match those of the cornea on which it will rest. In this case, consultation with an ophthalmologist rather than with an *optometrist* is particularly important, even though a contact lens technician associated with an ophthalmologist may do the actual fitting and instruction in contact lens care.

Not all ophthalmologists fit patients for contact lenses. If yours does not, ask him to refer you to an ophthalmologist who does, or you may prefer to find one yourself. The two best sources for this information are a department of ophthalmology at a nearby teaching hospital (at your request, the hospital will be able to give you the names of ophthalmologists on their staff who have private practices and fit contact lenses), and the Contact Lens Association of Ophthalmologists, a national organization of contact lens specialists. They, too, will be glad to furnish two or three names of doctors in your area. (See Appendix.)

Getting Fitted for Contact Lenses

Rigid Gas-Permeable Lenses

The fitting of rigid gas-permeable and soft lenses differs significantly, as do the insertion and removal procedures.

The rigid lens fitting begins with a complete eye examination, including a determination of the optical correction. Because rigid lenses must conform to the size and shape of the cornea (this is what ensures a comfortable fit), the shape of the cornea is measured with a special instrument called a keratometer.

Once these measurements have been taken, a pair of lenses is ordered from the laboratory, and the patient is asked to return for a second visit when the lenses are ready. At that time, the lenses will be inserted and checked for proper fit and optics. If everything is satisfactory, the patient is given detailed instructions in how to care for and

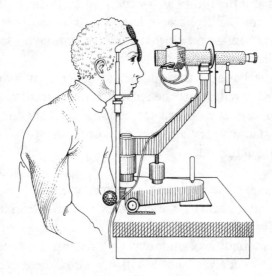

Fig. 4.6   A keratometer, used to measure the shape of the cornea

properly insert and remove the new lenses. Finally, the patient is put on a wearing schedule appropriate to individual needs and lens type so that all-day comfort is achieved.

Patients are seen once or twice a week during their initial adaptation period to keep track of their progress, to determine if there are any problems, and to answer any questions they may have.

Soft Lenses

The fitting for soft lenses begins with the same office visit and the same complete eye examination. The prescription for soft lenses, however, is less complicated than for hard ones. Although the optics of soft lenses vary as much, their softness and flexibility allow them to conform to the shape of the cornea. There are, in fact, only a handful of prescription variations—so few that a doctor can have a stock supply on hand.

On the basis of the optics and corneal measurements, your doctor will select the lens most likely to fit you, examine the lenses and optical correction, and if the findings are not satisfactory, try another pair until the perfect fit and optics are achieved.

Whichever type of lenses selected, contact lens wearers should have their eyes *and* lenses examined on a regular basis. Your doctor will schedule checkups, generally following a schedule of once every six months for lens checks, and once every year and a half for a complete eye examination. These checkups are particularly important because they allow your doctor to monitor the medical health of your eyes, especially the cornea. They are also of value because rigid lenses can become scratched or chipped in a way that could cause eye irritation or corneal injury, even though the wearer may notice nothing. Soft lenses may develop tears, nicks, or deposits that may also escape the wearer's notice.

Using Your Contact Lenses

You can rest assured that your contact lenses are completely safe as long as you follow three important rules. The first is that you get your lenses through a medical contact lens specialist, and the second is that you return for periodic checkups. The third is that you follow to the letter the doctor's instructions regarding the proper care and cleaning of the lenses, as well as for their hygienic insertion and removal. This third rule is too often not followed, for contact lenses—both rigid and soft—have strict requirements for their maintenance and use. Yet considering the many and great advantages of contacts over glasses, you will find that once you have become accustomed to following the drill, it will be an easily borne inconvenience.

Rigid Lenses

Rigid-lens patients are instructed to use the following technique: The safest way to clean your lenses is to first wash your hands thoroughly with soap and water to remove any irritating substances, such as nicotine or skin oils, which can cause discomfort. Rinse well to remove any oils or perfumes in the soap itself, then dry your hands on a lint-free towel. Do not try to insert or remove a lens over the sink. No matter how careful you are to close the drain, the one time you forget is inevitably the time you drop a lens. Even if it does not escape that way, a lens dropped on the sink or any other hard surface can become scratched, chipped, or warped.

Spread a clean towel over a flat surface. Place the cleaning and soaking solutions, one cup of lukewarm water, a standing mirror, and your contact lenses in their case on top of the towel. You will have to clean your lenses thoroughly before and after each wearing. This is not an overcautious measure that can be neglected from time to time. Contact lenses pick up particles from the air and other contaminants during wear, and lenses should not be returned to their case until they have been properly cleaned. In time, these substances can harden on the lens surface, making cleaning more difficult. The sooner the lenses are cleaned, the easier it is to do a good job of it. And although it may seem that the lenses should emerge from their case as clean as when you put them there, the case itself is not a perfectly sterile environment and the lenses may pick up contaminants and irritants even there.

Many lenses have a small dot or mark printed on the right lens to help you tell them apart. The dot is visible when the lens is out of the eye, but it cannot be noticed once the lens is in place. Whether or not lenses are marked in this way, it is a good idea always to start with the right lens; this makes it easier for you to remember which is which.

Hold the lens gently by the edges and apply a drop of cleaning solution to both sides. Rub the lens lightly between thumb and index finger to distribute the solution over the entire surface. Avoid using your fingernails, and do not apply pressure to the lens. Immerse the lens in the cup of water and rub gently to rinse off the cleaning solution, but do not attempt to dry it. Again holding the lens gently by the edges, apply a drop of wetting solution to each side. The lens is now ready to be inserted.

Place the lens concave side up on the tip of your moistened index finger, and with the middle finger of the same hand pull down the lower eyelid. Raise the other arm over your head and lift the upper eyelid with your middle or index finger—whichever is more comfortable and secure—by grasping the eyelid near the lash line. Look straight at the center of your lens (it is now in front of your eye and slightly below it). Keeping your finger on the eyelid, move the lens toward your eye until it makes contact

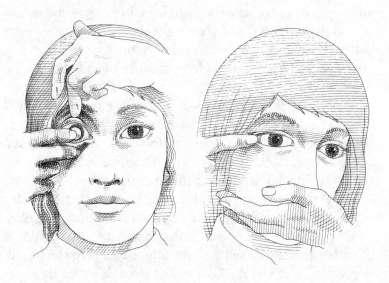

Fig. 4.7 Techniques for rigid contact lens insertion (left) and removal

with your cornea. At this point release your eyelid. Close your left eye to make sure that the vision in your right eye is good and that the lens is properly located. Repeat the same procedure for your left eye. The key to easy insertion is to stay relaxed, keep your eyes wide open, and stare straight ahead.

The removal technique begins with the same setup, whether you are taking out your lenses at the end of the day or you have a particle or irritant in your eye. There is no need to panic if you have something in your eye, and a hasty and careless emergency removal is one of the surest ways to lose a contact lens.

Once you have set up towel and lens paraphernalia and

have washed your hands thoroughly, lean over the towel and begin by removing the right lens. Place your index finger on the outer edge of your right eye, as close to the eyeball as possible, and pull the eyelid to the side while forcing your eyelids to stay open. Cup your other hand under your eye and then blink. The lens should fall out into your cupped hand. If it misses it will land on the towel, which is there as a soft-surface backup to protect your lens from being scratched. Sometimes the lens will adhere to your eyelashes or cheek, so before you panic and start searching the floor, check your face in the mirror.

Once you have located the lens, hold it gently by the edges and repeat the cleaning procedure outlined above. Then return the lens to its clean case, add some soaking solution, and close the case carefully. Make sure the lens is safely tucked in and the lid does not close down on its edge. Repeat these same steps for the left eye.

One danger of bacterial contamination arises from the foolish habit of using saliva as a wetting solution. Never do this. The mouth is one of the most bacteria-laden parts of the body, and although it is true that your eyes have certain natural bacteria, they are not the same as those found in your mouth. Spitting on a contact lens or wetting it with your tongue risks serious eye infection. If you ever find yourself without a bottled wetting solution designed for your type of lenses, use plain tap water. Wetting solution increases comfort temporarily, but it is quickly washed away by tears. Water is an acceptable substitute; saliva is most emphatically not.

Within a short time, lens handling will become an easy, routine matter. It should not, however, become a matter of carelessness. Strict adherence to these measures will ensure that the lenses stay in good condition and that you will be able to wear them with comfort.

Soft Lenses

The hygiene and insertion and removal procedures for soft lenses differ considerably from those for rigid lenses. The soft lens routine may seem more complicated, but here, too, you can quickly adjust to it and easily integrate the procedures into your daily schedule. The specific details vary, depending on the manufacturer of the soft lens in question, so your doctor should explain how best to use the lenses prescribed. There are some things that are generally true for all soft lenses, regardless of type.

The absorptive plastic that makes soft lenses flexible must not be allowed to dry out or to absorb anything other than the special solutions intended for use with the soft lenses. Neither rigid-lens solutions nor any other emergency substitutes should be used. Soft lenses are stored wet, and because they pick up bacteria and other irritants, special cleaning procedures are required.

Scrupulous hand washing and rinsing are essential before handling soft lenses.

When you are ready to put in your lenses, wash your hands well and set up a towel, mirror, your lens solution bottle, and lens case on a table. Carefully remove the right lens from the case and examine it to make sure it is moist and clean. Because they are flexible, soft lenses can be turned inside out. Check to be sure this has not happened on its own, and if it has, reverse the lens.

Clean the lens with the recommended solution. Place the lens in the palm of your hand, with the concave side up.

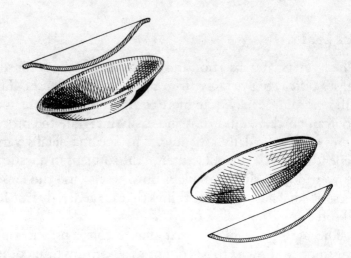

**Fig. 4.8   The soft contact lens on the left is inside out.
The one on the right is correct.**

Wet it with solution and rub the lens gently between your
thumb and index fingertips. Take care not to let the lens
touch your nails. The lens is now ready to be inserted.

Place the lens on the outer edge of your index finger,
using whichever hand is most comfortable. Hold your head
erect and gaze upward at the same time as you pull down
your lower eyelid with the middle finger of the same hand.
Keep your eyes fixed on a point above you, but do not move
your head up—the idea is to expose a larger portion of your
sclera below the cornea. Gently move the lens onto the
sclera, then remove your index finger and release the lower

eyelid. Close your eyes for a moment and the lens will center itself.

When you are ready to remove the lens, wash hands thoroughly and make sure they are well rinsed. Hold your head erect and gaze upward. Pull down the lower eyelid with your middle finger and put your index finger on the bottom edge of the lens. Gently, without exerting much pressure, slide the lens down onto the sclera. Once the lens is on the sclera, keep your index finger on the lens and continue gazing upward and holding down the lower eyelid. Place your thumb and index finger on either side of the lens

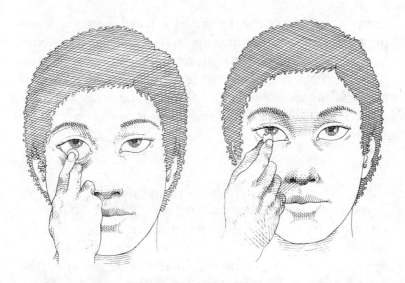

Fig. 4.9   Techniques for soft contact lens insertion (left) and removal (right)

and gently roll them together, pinching the lens so it doubles up between your fingers. This allows air to get under the lens, thus breaking the suction on your tear layer. Once you have the lens pinched between your fingers, remove it from your eye. Clean the lens again, return it to its case, and add some solution.

You can insert and remove soft lenses in one-tenth the time it takes to explain the procedure. If you take care to keep hands free of irritants and always work with lenses that are clean and of the right consistency, you can perform the entire technique deftly and comfortably.

Special Contact Lens Problems

In the past 40 years the sight of a panicked individual clapping hand to eye and running off to the nearest restroom has been a common one. Unfortunately, this has led many people to believe that contact lenses are fraught with danger and distress. But in fact, if proper precautions are taken, contact lenses can be safely and comfortably worn.

Chips and Scratches

Rigid lenses are vulnerable to scratching and chipping. Wearers may not notice minute flaws, but such flaws can cause irritation and obviously should be avoided. During your periodic checkups your doctor will examine lenses to determine if they are flawed in any way, but only the wearer can prevent them from becoming damaged. Avoid all hard surfaces: Do not touch your lenses with your fingernails, and if you wear rings, remove them before handling your contacts. Do not bounce your lenses around on mirrors and other hard surfaces. Take great care not to drop them. Rather, insert and remove them over a towel, not over the sink. Lenses will not become scratched through normal wear.

Replacing Lenses

If lenses are severely scratched or chipped, they will have to be replaced. But this is not something that will inevitably occur in the course of time—some patients wear their lenses faithfully for years and, because they take proper precautions, the lens surfaces remain as smooth as the day they were first fitted.

If you do lose a rigid lens, call your doctor so a replacement can be ordered immediately. It usually takes only a few days. Soft lenses are usually in stock, so replacement can be almost immediate. When traveling abroad, phone or cable your doctor and the lenses can be mailed within a few days. If you can afford it, the ideal solution would be to have a spare pair.

The two most common reasons for losing lenses need never occur: (1) A particle of dust enters the eye, causing momentary irritation and quick removal, and (2) the lens slips off the cornea onto the sclera. Do not panic in either case, and do not try to remove the lens outside or in the middle of a dance floor.

A Particle in the Eye

A particle will usually be washed out with the tears triggered by the irritation. If it is not, calmly and slowly make your way to a quiet corner where you can set up for removal. Do not stand over a restroom sink. Instead, lay a paper towel or handkerchief on a flat surface near a mirror, have the case and lens solution at hand, and proceed in the normal fashion.

Decentration

If the lens has slipped onto the sclera, it can remain there without doing any harm. Vision through that eye will be poor since it is no longer through the lens, but the eye cannot be damaged by a lens on the sclera for a short while. Soft lenses rarely get decentered, but rigid lenses sometimes do. If this happens, the situation can be rectified in one of three ways:

The first but least effective way is to look in a mirror, locate the lens, and then look in the direction of the lens. This brings the cornea toward the lens in an attempt to get the lens to recenter itself on the particular contours on which it was designed to float. If this does not work, close your eyes and gently massage the eyelid until the lens is back on the cornea. Do not press hard; exert only as much pressure as needed to move the lens gradually toward the cornea. The third method uses the index finger on the eyelid margin. Look in a mirror and move the eyelid (the bottom one if the lens is below the cornea; the top if it is above) to gently push the lens along until it regains its position on the cornea. Do not, in any circumstances, place your finger directly on the eyeball. Many times the lens will drop out of the eye in the midst of these procedures. When that happens, simply clean the lens, reapply wetting solution, and reinsert it. But be sure to work on a flat surface covered with a towel or soft cloth so the lens does not get scratched if it does pop out.

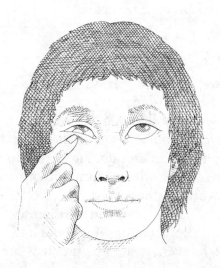

Fig. 4.10 Recentering a lens, using index finger and eye-lid margin

Discomfort

Some contact lens wearers, particularly soft-lens wearers, are disturbed by low levels of humidity, such as those that occur in overheated houses during the winter. The best solution is to add humidity to the air by opening a window, using a room humidifier, or turning down the heat. If this is not practical, moisturizing eyedrops can be used.

Glare can sometimes be a problem for contact lens wearers. Lightly tinted lenses reduce glare somewhat. For the outdoors, a pair of nonprescription sunglasses will cut glare. Sunglasses are also helpful on windy days, especially during the initial adjustment period, because they provide a shield against dust and airborne particles.

When Not to Wear Them

Contact lenses, rigid or soft, are designed to be worn throughout the waking day. Wearers can engage in any and all activities, regardless of how strenuous. In fact, lenses lend themselves to contact sports, dancing, and other such activities better than glasses do. However, doctors do not advise wearing lenses when swimming or bathing unless goggles are worn or the eyes are kept closed or closely squinted. Many people have lost their lenses this way—a contact lens that floats out of the eye and into a swimming pool is gone forever. If aerosol products are used, first remove your lenses. If this is not feasible, be sure to keep your eyes closed while you are spraying and for a minute or two afterward until no more spray remains in the air.

Finally, except for extended-wear types, contact lenses are not intended to be worn during sleep. Blinking is an important part of what makes contacts safe, and one does not blink when asleep.

A pair of well-fitting contact lenses, worn regularly and kept in good condition, will provide the best possible optical correction. Unlike glasses, which create a sort of triple optical system that can distort the size of viewed objects and therefore sometimes make it impossible to achieve 20/20 vision, contact lenses closely approximate nature's optical system. Their medical and nonmedical applications have made it possible for millions of people to see well and to maintain the health of their eyes. When fitted by or under the supervision of a medical eye doctor and cared for properly, they are a significant improvement over glasses, providing a far more natural window on the world.

Radial Keratotomy: A Postscript

In the blurry world of the nearsighted, the prospect of chucking one's eyeglasses forever is the stuff that dreams are made of. An eye operation called radial keratotomy done by a few ophthalmologists makes claims in this area. If the surgery proves a complete success, it promises the patient a quality of vision without glasses as good as it was with glasses.

Radial keratotomy was developed in 1974 by a Soviet surgeon named Fyodorov and subsequently embraced by a few U.S. ophthalmologists. It involves changing the shape of the cornea to alter its refractive (light-bending) power.

The surgeon makes anywhere from four to sixteen incisions, which radiate outward from the center of the cornea like the spokes of a wheel. As the cornea heals, it flattens out in the center. This flattening has the same effect as corrective lenses, changing the angle of light rays entering the eye. Ideally, that change will focus the rays directly on the retina, so that objects no longer look blurry.

The procedure is usually performed in two separate sessions—one for each eye—and can be done under local anesthesia. Postoperative pain is generally mild to moderate for a day or so, and vision is initially cloudy. But most patients are able to return to work in a few days and resume driving in a week.

Initial enthusiasm, especially in the media, helped create a lucrative new market.

During the last few years, however, more rigorous

assessments of the surgery have shed some sobering light on it.

Radial keratotomy is a procedure with very uncertain ramifications. It may reduce or eliminate the need for corrective lenses, but additional long-term data are sorely needed. Because the cornea takes approximately four to five years to heal fully after surgery, reliable long-term studies are not yet available. According to the American Academy of Ophthalmology, the benefits "must be weighed against the possibility of immediate or future impairment of sight or other complications."

The U.S. Air Force has decreed that no candidate for enlistment who has undergone radial keratotomy will be accepted. Many who have had the procedure report being bothered by glare at night, and they experience some fluctuations in their visual acuity. These problems would be particularly detrimental for military aviators.

But if the value and safety of the operation are questionable, why are doctors allowed to perform it? It is an anomaly in American medicine that allows wide latitude for surgical procedures. If a drug or implant were developed for nearsightedness, the U.S. Food and Drug Administration (FDA) would require extensive testing for safety and effectiveness before approving it. But any licensed M.D. is legally entitled to perform radial keratotomy in the United States. There are no supervisory or control procedures in place to prevent this.

On the plus side of radial keratotomy is that the great majority of patients will have improved optics, and many may indeed be able to discard their glasses even if their visual acuity is not 20/20.

It should be kept in mind, however, that this procedure involves operating on a healthy eye. At best, the operation will produce visual acuity that is no better than that already available with glasses or contact lenses. That makes it all the more important to weigh the potential benefits against the possible complications and outcome of surgery. These include infection, glare in the vision not present before, variability in visual acuity, and under- or overcorrection of the optical error. Furthermore, the procedure leaves small opaque scars on the cornea, a structure intended to be optically clear. Another potential problem is that the patient who still needs optical correction after the procedure may have difficulty wearing contact lenses on the reshaped and scarred cornea. That individual thus loses out on what is widely regarded as the overwhelmingly superior approach to the correction of optical errors.

About Cataracts

◇

MYTH: Cataracts can be surgically removed only when they are ripe.

FACT: A cataract is not a tomato and does not ripen like one. A cataract can worsen, but the time for surgery, if it is needed at all, is when vision is sufficiently impaired to interfere with daily life.

MYTH: Older people frequently develop second sight.

FACT: This so-called second sight is usually a developing cataract, which produces a tendency toward nearsightedness. The increasing nearsightedness permits artificially good vision of close objects and frequently makes it possible to read without glasses even though they were previously needed. This is *not* a good thing, since it indicates a developing cataract.

MYTH: Eyedrops and/or oral medication can prevent or slow cataracts.

FACT: There is no known treatment other than surgery for cataracts. Some studies have suggested that aspirin may slow cataract development, but a causal connection has not been satisfactorily established and the thesis remains highly speculative at this time.

Cataracts are the leading cause of blindness in the world. In fact, nearly 50 percent of all blindness can be traced to cataracts. But the vast majority of these cases are found in the Third World, where poor nutrition and inadequate medical care are important factors. In the United States, the senile cataract is the overwhelmingly most common type, and in most cases it is easily treated.

What Is a Cataract?

A cataract is any imperfection in the clarity of the lens of the eye, for whatever reason. Because the lens must be perfectly clear to allow light to pass through it on the way to the retina, an imperfection of this sort can affect sight. How much the effect on sight depends on the size and density of the imperfection, and that can vary greatly. If you think of the lens as a window, a cataract can be like a speck of dust that is easy to look past and ignore. Or it can be like a steamed-up window, which allows you to see only vague shapes and gradations in light and dark. It can also be like a window that has been painted black, through which you can see little if anything.

Cataracts also vary greatly in their effect on vision,

depending on where they are located on the lens. Whether a cataract is located in the front or back of the lens may have no effect on the degree of visual loss, but its location either in the center or near the periphery of the lens can make a big difference. If the clouding of the lens is at or near the visual axis (the center of the pupil), vision will be more greatly impaired. The more to the side of the lens the clouding is, the less severe the symptoms will be. Often the clouding is fairly equal throughout the lens.

Anatomy of the Lens

The lens of the eye is a remarkable structure. It usually is perfectly clear because no blood vessels enter or leave it. It gets its nutrition from the clear aqueous fluid it is bathed in. It has two functions: to refract (bend) rays of light as they enter the eye and to focus the light by changing shape and thickness. That ability to change shape and thickness is what enables the eye to focus from near objects to far ones and back again. In its incredible simplicity the lens is almost as magical as the extremely complicated eye itself.

As in so many of nature's great designs, the anatomy of the lens is rather simple. The lens is totally surrounded by a capsule. Under the front (anterior) portion of the capsule is a specialized layer of cells, which reproduce and become lens fibers.

Lens fibers are produced throughout life, with new ones being laid down over the old. The fibers in the center of the lens are compressed together and form a compact mass called the *nucleus.* The lens increases slightly in size each time a layer is added. Over time, the layers become increas-

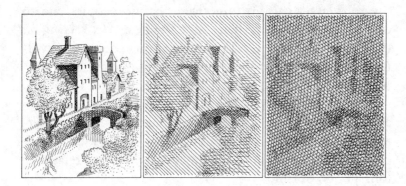

Fig. 5.1 Cataracts can affect vision in various ways: *(left)* vision with an early or minimal cataract can be close to normal; *(center)* vision as a cataract becomes more advanced can be fairly blurred; *(right)* vision with a severe cataract can be extremely blurred.

ingly compressed, making the lens material more rigid. Late in life this process tends to make the lens less clear.

Depending on the extent and density of the lens disclarity, cataracts can be symptomless or they can have extremely subtle or very obvious symptoms. In all cases, however, the symptoms have to do with how well you see, since in no case does a cataract cause pain, excessive tearing, redness, or any other eye discomfort. If the cataract is of the "specks on the window" type, no visual problem will be experienced. Patients with more extensive cataracts invariably come to their doctors requesting new glasses because things seem less clear to them and the resolution of images is less sharp than it used to be. Very often, however, even a severe cataract can go unnoticed because people tend to compensate for diminished vision in one eye by relying on the other, stronger eye. This is something people do involuntarily; they are rarely aware of using one eye predominantly. There may be some loss of depth perception because only one eye is delivering a sharp message, but this is usually too slight to be noticed in normal, daily use. Furthermore, cataracts in most cases develop very gradually, so people adjust to the subtle changes in sight over a relatively long period of time.

Types of Cataracts

Senile Cataracts

By far the most common cause of cataracts is simply advancing age; this is the so-called *senile cataract.* Because the lens grows throughout life, adding new cell layers to the outside periphery in a way similar to the growth rings of a tree, its size, resiliency, and clarity undergo change. The lens gets somewhat larger, but the major changes affect resiliency and clarity, because the layers are compacted and the lens tends to get more rigid and less transparent later in life. This process occurs in everyone's eyes as a natural result of aging, although the rate of change obviously varies among individuals. The rigidity contributes to the loss of focusing ability we call presbyopia; the decreased transparency causes a cataract.

Congenital Cataracts

A much rarer type of cataract, the *congenital cataract,* is present at birth. It is caused by some event during fetal development at the time the eye is formed. One of the known causes of congenital cataracts is exposure to the rubella (German measles) virus in the first trimester of pregnancy.

Secondary Cataracts

Secondary cataracts are cataracts caused by something other than the aging process or by an insult during the prenatal period. One type often seen in Third World countries results from a diet deficient in protein, and thus it is called a *nutritional cataract.*

Other secondary cataracts are brought about by internal eye infections. Any infection in the anterior chamber or in the vitreous fluid, whatever its cause, increases the likelihood of cataract formation.

Medications may also cause cataracts. One of the most common is the corticosteroid group of drugs, often used in the treatment of arthritis and other inflammatory conditions. The longer the drug is used and the higher the dosage, the more likely it is that a secondary cataract will form.

Traumatic cataract results from a blow to the eye. If the blow is severe enough and angled correctly, it may impair the functioning of the lens either by displacing it or by interfering with its metabolism. A penetrating wound that directly hits the lens will invariably cause a cataract.

An imbalance of body chemicals or hormones may cause a *metabolic cataract.* The most common example of this is a diabetic cataract. A rarer one results from low thyroid function (hypothyroidism).

Secondary cataracts may be caused by radiation exposure, whether accidental (a faulty microwave oven, perhaps) or from cancer therapy or other medical treatments. Here again, the dosage and frequency levels are the key.

Certain chemicals can cause secondary cataracts if they are absorbed at above-normal levels. Naphthalene, the active ingredient in mothballs, is one example, although the amount contained in mothballs is not great enough to damage the eye.

Finally, a high-voltage electrical shock to the body can cause a secondary cataract.

An Ancient Affliction

Cataracts have been recognized since Roman times, and one of the earliest depictions of cataract surgery can be seen in a second-century Roman bas relief. The procedure, called *couching,* was used until the eighteenth century. The lens is not removed from the eye, but instead a needle is inserted into the eye and used in an attempt to dislocate the lens. If the attempt is successful, the lens is pushed out of the central axis so it no longer interferes with vision and falls back into the vitreous fluid. Technically, if all went well and there was no infection, the procedure could work.

The first description of a *cataract extraction* (removal of the lens from the eye) is from the mid-eighteenth century. Lack of anesthesia and a high infection rate made the procedure both extremely painful and extremely risky at first. In the nineteenth century, however, with the development of anesthesia and antisepsis, results improved. In the twentieth century, a variety of new procedures have been developed, most of them contributing in an important way to greater safety. Today cataract surgery has become among the safest and most effective of all surgical procedures.

The words *cataract* and *cataract surgery* inspire anxiety and wishful denial in most people, primarily because so many are ignorant of the facts about cataracts and eye surgery in general. It is an unavoidable though hardly pleasant fact that the majority of us who are fortunate enough to live to a ripe old age will develop cataracts, for indeed the most common type of cataract is part of the natural process of aging. But it is also true that having a cataract does not automatically mean surgery. If surgery is needed, the cataract operation is extremely safe and remarkably effective, and sight can be corrected after surgery to provide a far better picture of the world than was possible before the cataract was removed.

If You Have a Cataract

◇

MYTH: Cataracts can grow back after surgery.
FACT: Cataracts are a clouding of the lens of the eye, and because the lens is removed in all types of cataract surgery, neither the cataract nor the lens can grow back.

MYTH: When you have cataract surgery, your eyeball is removed from the socket and then replaced after the operation is over.
FACT: No eye surgery involves removal of an eyeball from its socket. When cataract surgery is performed, an incision is made in the front of the eyeball to give access to the lens of the eye. This is easily done without dislocating the eyeball.

MYTH: There is a new method of cataract surgery that uses laser beams.
FACT: Laser beams are never used to remove cataracts.

People who believe this are probably thinking of *phakoemulsification,* a cataract surgical technique that uses a needlelike instrument to suction out the lens of the eye. A laser may be used to destroy a membrane, which may be a complication resulting from previous cataract surgery.

Ophthalmologists are trained as medical doctors, and as such they are qualified to deal with any and all pathologies of the eye, as well as refractive errors. Optometrists are licensed and trained to diagnose refractive errors and treat nonmedical problems with corrective glasses or contact lenses. Optical errors—deviations from optimal vision at the site where images are focused in relation to the retina—are not diseases, any more than having arms too short to scratch your back is a disease.

When it comes to the treatment of cataracts, the difference between optometrists and ophthalmologists is extremely important to understand. Ophthalmologists are certainly the only one of these two eye specialists qualified to recommend and apply surgical remedies.

If you have a cataract, the first time you become aware of it will probably be when your ophthalmologist tells you about it. In all likelihood you will not yet have noticed any change in your vision. You may have friends and relatives who have cataracts and who still see reasonably well. You may know that some of these people live with cataracts and that others have had them surgically removed. Cataracts that come with aging are quite common, but the subject remains one in which there is a great deal of misinformation. Knowing what to expect if you are told you have cataracts can help diminish much of the anxiety and stress usually associated with such a diagnosis. If you do learn that you have cataracts, your experience will probably be similar to that of the patient described below.

The Diagnosis

When Linda A, a 63-year-old free-lance editor, arrived for her annual checkup, the doctor reviewed her chart and noted that she was slightly nearsighted in her right eye but had not required glasses for distance viewing. At her age she had, of course, lost near-focusing ability in both eyes (see chapter 3).

In the examining room, she mentioned that on occasion her vision did not seem quite as sharp as it once had been. She wondered whether she might possibly need some correction for distance vision.

While conducting a complete eye examination using dilating drops and examining the interior of her eyes through the biomicroscope, the ophthalmologist observed that she had developed early senile cataracts in both eyes. The cataract in her right eye was slightly more severe than the one in her left. These early cataracts were responsible for her suspicion that her distance vision was not as sharp as it used to be.

In her right eye, the cataract limited her best possible corrected vision to 20/40; her slight refractive error decreased it to 20/50, but that additional ten points could be corrected with glasses. Her left eye was without refractive error, although the less advanced cataract limited her vision to 20/25. By prescribing stronger reading glasses the doctor could provide her a little added magnification in near-viewing situations, allowing slightly better resolution to compensate for the mild cataracts. In this way her near (reading) vision could be corrected to 20/30 in the right eye and nearly 20/20 in the left. The difference between the two eyes was small enough and the overall visual acuity good enough to be easily tolerable.

Aside from the cataracts, Ms. A's medical eye examination was perfectly normal. There were no signs of other medical eye problems: Her intraocular pressure was normal, as were her retina, cornea, and eye muscles.

Because the cataract was causing noticeable vision problems, Ms. A had to be told. If the cataract were so small as to have no practical effect, and if the patient could be depended on to have regular medical eye checkups, the ophthalmologist might decide to say nothing. However, many doctors today believe that patients have the right to know all the doctor's findings no matter how inconsequential. If you are over 50 and you want to know the precise findings of any examination, simply ask if there is any evidence of cataracts. Your doctor will always answer such a direct question truthfully.

Because the eyes frequently reflect general health problems, and some of these problems may contribute to the development of cataracts or influence how they are managed, the ophthalmologist asked, among other questions, if Ms. A suffered from diabetes, high blood pressure, anemia, or kidney problems. Cataracts, for example, are much more common in diabetics than in the general population, and poorly controlled diabetes can accelerate their growth. The physician also inquired about any medications Ms. A might be taking, particularly steroids, which could also accelerate the growth of cataracts. Ms. A assured her physician that her last physical, three months before, showed her to be in good health.

Although distance glasses would improve sight in her

right eye ever so slightly, they would be of insufficient benefit to warrant their use. But the doctor recommended stronger reading glasses because Ms. A needed optimal vision for her editorial work.

Ms. A was told that the cataract she had—by far the most common type—was referred to as "senile," but that this had nothing to do with senility. The name reflects its relationship to the aging process. Almost everyone who is fortunate enough to get old will probably develop this type of cataract.

The doctor explained that her cataracts might stabilize or worsen but that they would not improve. No change in reading or work habits would accelerate or slow down their rate of development. She might see more clearly, however, if she worked and read in a brightly lit area, and a lamp equipped with a halogen bulb was recommended.

Ms. A was asked to return for a reevaluation in six months instead of a full year. If she noticed any problems with her vision, she was instructed to come sooner.

The doctor reassured Ms. A that it was far too soon to discuss surgery, although present-day cataract surgery is one of the safest and most restorative of surgical procedures. In fact, she might never need surgery, and if she ever did, the type would depend both on her condition and the ophthalmological procedures available at that time.

Six Months Later

When Ms. A returned for her scheduled checkup, she reported that her new reading glasses were helpful, that she had noticed little additional change in her eyes, but that she felt that night driving was slightly more difficult. The doctor was not surprised to hear this complaint, as it is one of the first voiced by people with developing cataracts. Lower light levels (hence poorer resolution), combined with the tension many people naturally feel when driving, is responsible. In addition, the haloing effect of headlights viewed through the slightly clouded lens of one's eye is unsettling to some drivers.

Once again Ms. A's pupils were dilated and her eyes examined under the biomicroscope. The examination revealed no progression of her cataracts. Her vision, both distance and near, was stable.

She was asked to return again in six months, and this she did regularly for the next several years.

Five Years Later

Ms. A was now 68 years old and still doing editing, although no longer full-time. When she had her regular six-month checkup, she reported a definite decrease in her vision, especially in her right eye.

When her vision was tested, the right eye's best correction for the distance was 20/80; the best correction in the left eye was still 20/25. The best corrected reading vision was still almost 20/20 in the left eye, although now 20/60 in the right.

Examining the eyes under the biomicroscope, the doctor observed greater clouding of the right cataract than had been seen previously.

Ms. A was now told that her right eye was far enough along to make cataract surgery a legitimate consideration, although by no means a necessity. Her left eye, however, was definitely not a candidate for surgery. The doctor explained that most people are usually not aware of the poorer vision in the more affected eye because the brain naturally selects the optically superior image.

Ms. A was assured that using her left eye more in compensation would not accelerate cataract growth or have any effect on the progress of the cataract in either eye. Nevertheless, the left eye might worsen on its own and that was a possibility to consider.

If Ms. A had surgery on the right eye and the left eye were to suddenly deteriorate, the right eye would have already been corrected. However, cataract development patterns generally continue as they have, so that the sudden worsening of a slowly developing cataract is unlikely. If Ms. A also had primary simple glaucoma (elevation of pressure inside the eye) in the same eye, it might be worth operating sooner, since it is a relatively simple matter during cataract surgery to do an additional procedure that treats glaucoma.

Cataracts sometimes cause a rare secondary glaucoma by mechanically interfering with the drainage of aqueous fluid. If that were the case, surgery would be medically indicated and removal of the lens in itself would most likely solve the secondary problem.

Sometimes a cataractous lens begins to soften as the nucleus undergoes degenerative changes. Because this may make surgery technically more difficult, such cataracts should be removed sooner rather than later.

The patient's general health is the next consideration. Severe, poorly controlled diabetes and hypertension, for example, bring with them a greater tendency for the eye to hemorrhage during surgery. This might influence a surgeon to delay cataract removal, at least until the diabetes or hypertension was better controlled.

Barring these and other unusual circumstances, the indication for surgery is visual loss, pure and simple. The patient should decide if cataract surgery is necessary for the successful functioning of his or her eyes. An elderly retired person with a moderate degree of visual loss may not be inconvenienced by the problem and therefore can do without surgery. That same visual loss in a 55-year-old architect would be a great handicap and therefore necessitate surgery. The decision about surgical correction should always be made based on a careful and thoughtful consideration of the patient's visual needs as well as the ophthalmologist's findings.

Since Ms. A's eyes were healthy and her general health good, her decision about surgery at this time was based primarily on comfort, bearing in mind that all surgery, no matter how safe, still carried some risk. It was agreed that she would defer surgery for the present, but that the cataracts would be reevaluated every four months instead of six.

Three Years Later

Ms. A, now age 71, was no longer active as an editor, but she did read a great deal in her increased spare time. Returning for a four-month examination, she related increased difficulty in reading. The examination revealed a best corrected-distance vision of 20/200 in her right eye and 20/40 in her left. Her near vision with reading glasses was a quite good 20/30 in the left eye, 20/80 in the right. The balance of her ophthalmological examination continued to be normal.

In the consultation room, Ms. A was informed that the time to operate on her right eye had probably arrived. Not only had the cataract in that eye continued to worsen, but the one in the left eye had begun to show changes as well. The doctor stressed that it was not a medical emergency; waiting longer would not threaten the ultimate health of her eyes. Still, he would ideally prefer to do surgery on her right eye and give it time to recover before Ms. A began to experience substantial visual loss in her left eye. In this way, a period of real visual disability could be avoided. The decision to go ahead with surgery, and the actual timing of the procedure, ultimately remained with the patient.

Considering Surgery

The doctor explained that he preferred to do cataract surgery in the hospital. Ms. A would go in on the day of the surgery and return home the same evening. Most ophthalmologists do cataract surgery as an outpatient procedure, with the patient spending a few hours resting in a recovery area before going home, but some ophthalmologists feel it is slightly safer to do it in a hospital, with at least an overnight stay. If any problems arise in the immediate postoperative period, they can be dealt with promptly, and 24 hours of supervised rest is a conservative precaution. However, Medicare and some insurance companies now insist on no overnight stay, barring complications.

Because it is safer than general anesthesia, most ophthalmologists prefer local anesthesia. Individuals in poor general health, especially those with cardiac or respiratory problems or the extreme elderly, are generally not good candidates for general anesthesia. If, however, a patient is extremely nervous or is mentally disabled, or for any reason is unable to cooperate during the procedure, and no health problems weigh against it, general anesthesia will be used.

The Case for an Implant

Because Ms. A's eyes were healthy, an intraocular lens implant was advised. Although the implant adds slightly to the risk of the procedure (it involves, after all, inserting a foreign body into the eye and leaving it there), most doctors feel that the risk-to-benefit ratio in a healthy eye warrants its use. In addition, the ratio becomes less favorable when an individual has glaucoma or diabetes. With glaucoma, the presence of the implant might further interfere with the delicate balance within the eye, so that an intracapsular extraction and externally worn contact lens might be preferable. With diabetics, who have a greater risk of severe bleeding during eye surgery, the more extensive implant procedure might slightly increase the risk of hemorrhage.

What to Expect After the Operation

Removal of the natural lens causes extreme farsightedness because the primary light-bending structure in the eye is removed (the cornea remains), leaving the image well out of focus when it reaches the retina. The refractive power formerly provided by the natural lens must be restored in at least one of the following ways: A lens implant is put in place during surgery; the patient is fitted with contact lenses; or the doctor prescribes glasses. In situations like Ms. A's, however, glasses are not a viable option. A high degree of magnification would be required to correct the farsight-

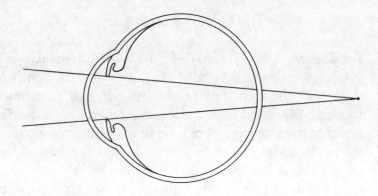

Fig. 6.1 Farsightedness caused by removal of a cataractous lens

edness in her right eye, but her unoperated left eye would see an image at normal size. The difference between the two would be intolerably disorienting (see chapter 4).

This shortcoming of the triple optical system (lens/air/ eye) does not occur with contact lenses, which rest directly on the tear layer of the eye and therefore present to each eye an image of unaltered size. If it were decided not to do an intraocular implant in her case, Ms. A could be fitted for a contact lens after the operation. For most people, this is the best alternative to an intraocular implant. A contact lens over the right eye will not create an incompatibility with the unoperated left eye. In some respects, this arrangement even has advantages: Its optical correction would correct for postoperative vision rather than relying on measurements for the implant taken prior to the operation. It should be mentioned that the optics of the lens implant cannot be changed after surgery.

Furthermore, an external contact lens will automatically correct any astigmatism that may have developed postoperatively as a result of sutures pulling unevenly on the cornea in the course of healing.

It should be noted here that even if any imprecision in the implant measurements before surgery were to make a postoperative optical correction necessary, the correction required would in all likelihood be too small to cause problems of image-size difference.

The Surgical Recommendation

Because there were no ophthalmological or general medical contraindications in Ms. A's case, as well as the fact that she had never worn contact lenses, the doctor recommended an intraocular lens implant for her. She had never worn contact lenses, and having an implant would mean that after the operation she would not have to go through an adjustment to wearing contacts. In all probability, she would be able to get about in the middle of the night or at any time during the day without any additional optical correction.

At the present time the surgical risk of the implant procedure is approximately 2 percent greater than cataract removal without implant, reducing the 98-percent success rate to about 96 percent. If the eye is healthy and the patient is over age 50, the slightly greater risk of the implant procedure is probably warranted. The benefit of having restoration of near normal vision without contact lenses or glasses generally outweighs the slightly added risk. With a patient who has worn contact lenses easily for years, however, the doctor would discuss not using an implant, relying instead on the contact lens to make the refractive correction.

Most doctors do not recommend a lens implant for patients under 45 simply because implants have not been around long enough for us to know how they will perform after 20 or 25 years, and young patients may be expected to live that long or longer.

It is possible for a patient to have the nonimplant procedure and, if dissatisfied, have a lens implanted at a later date. But this is among the poorest of choices, necessitating a second operation virtually as extensive as the original cataract procedure itself.

Having a lens implant in one eye and not the other creates no special problems except that a contact lens must be worn on the eye without the implant so that there is no dramatic difference in image size from one eye to the other. If and when the second eye needs cataract surgery, the decision to have an implant can be made anew for that eye, taking into account whether the patient was satisfied or dissatisfied with the earlier decision.

Ms. A was advised to obtain a second opinion if she had any doubts about her eye doctor's recommendation or if her insurance company required it before elective surgery, which this is. If she chose to get a second opinion, she would be advised to seek a board-certified ophthalmologist, preferably one associated with a teaching institution and one who was not connected professionally with her doctor.

Preliminaries

Six weeks later, Ms. A informed her doctor that she had sought a second opinion and had decided to go ahead with the cataract operation on her right eye. Ms. A and her doctor scheduled the surgery and arranged for preoperative screening, making it possible for her to be admitted on the day of surgery.

Ms. A's personal physician was informed of the intended cataract surgery so that the doctor could confirm that there was no aspect of her general health that might make surgery inadvisable at this time. The most common general health concern is uncontrolled high blood pressure, since it increases the risk of severe bleeding during eye surgery. Aspirin taken regularly (for arthritis, for example) also adds to the risk. This and other medications that might compromise surgery should be adjusted or, if possible, discontinued temporarily.

Two weeks before her scheduled surgery, Ms. A went to the hospital for preadmission tests. These included blood chemistry and blood count, urinalysis, an electrocardiogram, and a chest X ray. The entire battery of tests took less than half an hour, and the results were sent both to her ophthalmologist and to her personal physician.

Ms. A now had another eye examination, which found her eyes essentially unchanged. An A-scan, a painless examination that tells the doctor the optical strength of the intraocular lens implant to be ordered, was done. Her eyes were dilated, and it took just a few minutes for the specialized computer to make the measurement. The accuracy of A-scans is improving and now can determine the postoperative optics of an eye within a very acceptable range.

Because Ms. A's surgery was scheduled for about 9:30

A.M., she had to be at the hospital by 7:00 A.M. to register and get her preoperative medications. To minimize the possibility of vomiting, she was told to eat nothing after 9:00 P.M. the night before and to drink nothing, not even water, after midnight.

The Surgery

At the hospital Ms. A presented her insurance forms to the registration office, filled out her registration forms, and was taken to the outpatient waiting area. Shortly before 8:00 A.M., her ophthalmologist stopped by to say hello and to reassure her.

At about 8:15 she was given a surgical gown to put on and asked to lie on the stretcher on which she would be taken to the operating room. At about 8:30 the nurse administered injections into her buttocks and instilled dilating eyedrops; more eyedrops were administered at 9:00. The injections are usually a combination of a painkiller, sedative, and antinausea medications. She began to feel drowsy after 15 minutes or so but was definitely awake, a bit too nervous to go to sleep.

At a little after 9:00 A.M., an orderly wheeled her stretcher to a corridor outside the operating room. Fifteen minutes later, a nurse wheeled her into the operating room. Lying flat on her back, Ms. A saw stainless steel tables, cabinets, and shelves; white tile walls; and finally her doctor's face above her.

She was asked to move from the stretcher to the operating table and again lie flat on her back. She did this on her own, and a nurse placed a small ringlike pillow under her head to elevate and stabilize it. Her view was now of very bright overhead lights and green-masked faces moving about, mumbling instructions to one another.

Sterile drapes were placed over her body up to her nose and around her head. A small oxygen tube strapped under her nose and a metal lift that holds the drapes up permitted her to breathe comfortably. The skin around her eye was scrubbed to sterilize the area. For the third time, dilating drops were put into her right eye. By now her pupils were very widely dilated, a process that is best done gradually. The series of dilating drops guarantees a very large pupil, making access to the lens easier.

The drops contained a local anesthetic, so Ms. A's eye became somewhat numb, blocking sensation on the eyeball surface itself. The operation was done under local anesthesia. Ms. A was told that she would feel some needle sticks at the site of her bony orbit and in the joints of her upper and lower jaws as more anesthesia was administered by injection. These injections effectively paralyzed her upper and lower eyelids.

Ms. A was instructed to look up and far to the left as one final injection was administered. This went into the orbit, into the back of the eyeball. Besides blocking pain during the surgery, this local anesthesia also prevented Ms. A from squeezing her eyelids together or moving her eyeball while the surgery was in progress. A lid clamp that holds the eyelids apart further ensured an open field for surgery.

The Surgical Procedure

When the operation was ready to start, Ms. A was instructed to try to sleep. For the next hour or so she occasionally drifted into sleep, but most of the time she was just very relaxed and groggy. She had an awareness of low voices, the occasional low-volume sound of an instrument or machine, and of motion and activity around her eye.

The most common cataract operation performed in the United States today is called *extracapsular cataract extraction.* In this procedure, the posterior capsule (rear membrane) of the lens is left intact. This affords protection to the front of the vitreous fluid, keeping it from spilling forward and possibly having some vitreous fluid lost during surgery. It also permits less change of pressure on the retina and related structures in the back of the eye, thus decreasing the risk of such complications as retinal detachment and a cystlike swelling of the macula. On the other hand, leaving behind any other lens material, in this case the posterior capsule, runs the risk that it will turn opaque, in effect forming what is called a secondary cataract. The retained lens material also increases the likelihood of postoperative infection and inflammation.

The operation performed on Ms. A was an extracapsular cataract extraction with a lens implant. It began as a bright light and an operating microscope were moved into position after the area around the eye was sterilized. The surgeon sat at the head of the operating table, just behind the top of the patient's head, and looked down through the microscope.

Using surgical scissors, the surgeon made an incision in the conjunctiva where it attached to the cornea and peeled back the conjunctiva from the sclera, revealing the place where the sclera and cornea meet. A surgical knife was then used to make a groove in the sclera at that juncture for about 11 millimeters (say, an area between 10:30 and 1:30 on a clock). This marked the intended incision.

The incision was made through the sclera along the full

length of the groove, giving access to the anterior chamber of the eyeball. A viscous fluid was then squirted into the anterior chamber through a fine needle. This filler material deepens the anterior chamber, which tends to collapse a bit when the incision is made.

To minimize the possibility of postoperative secondary glaucoma, a small triangular piece was cut from the outside of the iris. Called a *peripheral iridectomy,* this provided an additional passage for drainage between posterior and anterior chambers.

The lens itself was removed in parts. First, a portion of the anterior capsule (the front membrane) of the lens was removed. This was followed by the nucleus of the lens, the oldest and hardest central core. Next was the cortex, the softer, newer, more viscous portion of the lens, which surrounds the nucleus.

The posterior capsule (back membrane), which was left intact, was cleaned with an irrigating solution to flush out remnants of lens material and prepare it for the intraocular lens.

The lens implant, which is made of inert plastic, was now inserted into the posterior chamber, resting between the posterior capsule in back, and the back of the iris in front. It was held in place by spring loops.

The sclera and cornea were brought back together with tiny stitches. One or more of the stitches might have been partially put in place earlier. The incision in the conjunctiva would be closed either with a single suture or sealed by heat cautery.

Finally, the surgeon instilled medications to keep the pupil dilated and to prevent infection and reduce inflammation. Then the doctor patched the eye.

Ms. A had napped during the procedure, not sure of how

Posterior chamber lens implant

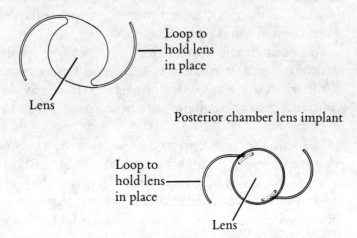

Lens

Loop to
hold lens
in place

Posterior chamber lens implant

Loop to
hold lens
in place

Lens

Two types of posterior chamber lens implants

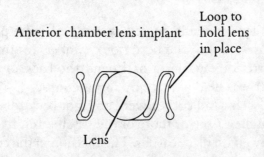

Anterior chamber lens implant

Loop to
hold lens
in place

Lens

Intraocular lens implants

Fig. 6.2

much time was spent asleep or awake. When she was slightly aroused by the sound of movement, she was told the operation was over and that all had gone well. Less than an hour had passed.

Recovery

Ms. A was taken back to the recovery room, with her eye bandaged, and was reminded to stay in bed until seen by the ophthalmologist and to ring for the nurse if she needed to go the bathroom. Emotionally drained and still under the effects of the medication, she fell asleep.

Around noontime, Ms. A's doctor awakened her and assured her again that all had gone well. She was advised to rest, go to the bathroom as necessary, and not to hesitate to ask for nursing help. Pain and sleeping medication were available upon request.

The doctor promised to return later, and if all appeared well she would be allowed to go home.

Before leaving, the doctor informed Ms. A that she might eat or drink anything she wished.

After drinking some juice, Ms. A fell asleep and awakened with some discomfort in midafternoon. She took some medication to relieve her pain.

Ms. A left the hospital early that evening, having already arranged for her daughter to take her home and stay with her overnight, at least for the first night or two.

Pain after cataract surgery is generally quite minimal, but it is variable from patient to patient. The patch on the eye tends to minimize pain, because the eye is forced closed under the patch; hence the patient avoids any blinking that would cause the eyelids to rub over the cornea. Once the patch is removed, blinking can be a source of pain. Any break in the corneal surface, loose sutures, or suture ends (not technically a surgical problem) can cause pain as the eye blinks. In cataract surgery the conjunctiva, the corneo-scleral junction, and the iris, all of which have nerve endings, are cut. The irritation of these nerves can cause some pain until the wound is healed. This becomes less and less likely as healing progresses after the operation. Pain can be mild and fairly steady or momentarily quite severe. Severe, constant pain is an extreme rarity.

Postoperative Care

Ms. A saw the doctor in his office the next day. After the bandage was removed, the eye and eyelid area were cleaned of discharge with sterile gauze and an irrigating solution. The doctor examined the eye with a bright light, an oph-thalmoscope, and a biomicroscope. The eye was still quite dilated, so in addition to a scratchy sore feeling with a lot of teariness, it was light-sensitive.

Ms. A asked the doctor to cover her good eye so she could look out of the operated one alone. She was disappointed that things looked very blurry but was reassured by her doctor that this was a normal postoperative reaction.

Before repatching her eye, the doctor put some medication into the eye. More dilating drops were included because a dilated eye is more at rest. The doctor also administered antibiotic drops or ointment to guard against external infections. Sometimes cortisone drops or ointment are used to minimize tissue reactions.

Ms. A was told she should avoid strenuous activity, walk slowly and carefully to avoid bumping her head, and remain at home until she came to the office. Any trauma to the freshly operated eye area would be undesirable because it could adversely affect healing, even possibly opening the wound. A jolt could cause intraocular complications, such as hemorrhage, lens-implant displacement, or even retinal detachment. Ms. A was given a prescription for mild anti-pain medication and a second prescription to help her sleep.

At home she read and watched television, using the unoperated left eye, the one she had used the most prior to her surgery anyway. She had a healthy appetite and slept well without any medication.

The next day, Ms. A's daughter brought her to the doctor's office again. The doctor removed the shield and bandage and examined the operated eye. Again, there was no evidence of complications. Ms. A remarked that the eye still felt scratchy and sore, but her vision seemed a bit clearer.

The doctor prescribed eyedrops to be used daily in the operated eye during this healing period and showed her how to apply the drops without pressing on her eye: Looking into a mirror, she was to pull down the lower eyelid, pushing only on the bone under the eyelid, not on the eyeball itself. This would expose the sac of the lower eyelid, where a drop of the medication should be placed. Ms. A was to take care not to touch the applicator tip to the eyeball or inner lid.

The doctor then showed Ms. A how to reattach the metallic shield with vertical strips of surgical paper tape, which pulls off the skin without any discomfort. She was instructed to continue to wear the shield all day and night for the time being.

Ms. A was given an appointment to return in three days. In the meantime she was told she could go out as much as she liked, use her eyes all she desired, but continue to avoid strenuous activity for about three to four weeks. She should particularly guard against bending over or bumping her forehead. She was told that she could take the pain and/or sleeping pills if necessary.

Two days later, four full days after surgery, Ms. A experienced a short-lived but fairly severe pain in her right eye. She called the doctor immediately and was told this was not unusual. The doctor suspected it was an irritation from one of the stitches, which might be pressing on a nerve, but to reassure them both she was told to come to the office that day so the eye could be examined. The examination showed normal healing, and the doctor confirmed that it was a suture causing the transient pain.

At her next visit, three days later, Ms. A reported needing no pain medication and feeling quite well. On examination, the eye appeared less red. Teariness and discharge were reduced, as was light sensitivity. The doctor obtained an uncorrected vision of 20/60. By experimentally holding a selection of lenses in front of that eye, the doctor was able to improve the vision to 20/40. It was explained that the eye was still healing, and the optics were still in flux. The cornea had been traumatized by the surgery and was somewhat swollen. It would be a while before her vision stabilized.

The doctor reassured Ms. A that the redness of her eye was normal and should be expected a week after surgery. The amount of discharge was also normal and did not indicate infection.

She was shown how to clean her eyelids herself now. Using the sterile irrigating solution and the small sterile gauze pads she was given, she was told to apply very little pressure, gently wiping the eyelid margins and corners— wherever there was crusted or moist discharge. She was instructed to do this once a day.

Ms. A was told to continue her daily drops but to wear the protective shield only while sleeping. She was to return in five days.

When seen again, 12 days after surgery, Ms. A said her eye felt quite comfortable, with only an occasional scratchy feeling. It looked almost as white as the other one and her vision had definitely cleared.

The examination revealed a well-healing eye with slightly less than 20/40 vision, correctable to almost 20/20 with an external lens. But since the eye was still healing, and its optical condition could change, the doctor did not want to prescribe corrective lenses. Until stabilized readings on two consecutive visits were obtained, the doctor preferred to make no determination about whether or not Ms. A would need glasses.

She was asked to return in one week and told to stop using the drops but to keep wearing the shield at night.

Corrected Vision

In the course of the next two examinations over a period of two weeks, the doctor observed that Ms. A's eye was healing well. Two consecutive stable readings of the vision in her right eye were obtained: 20/40 with the implant only, improvable to 20/20 with glasses. Her left eye, which had a developing cataract, a best corrected distance vision of 20/40, and a near vision of 20/30 prior to surgery, was unchanged. Inasmuch as her right eye could now improve its visual acuity, surpassing that which the left eye could achieve in its present state, glasses were recommended.

Together, Ms. A and her doctor discussed the option of two separate pairs of glasses, one for reading and one for distance, or bifocals for the sake of convenience. Several factors needed to be weighed. Ms. A had never worn bifocals before and thus would have to get used to them. She was no longer working, so the convenience of bifocals was not an important factor. Furthermore, she did not need distance glasses all the time. It was finally agreed that she would try two separate pairs: one for driving, watching television, or whenever she wanted optimal distance vision, and the second for reading and other near-distance situations.

The doctor advised her that now she could stop wearing the protective shield completely and resume all activities at a normal pace. She should still return for an examination every two weeks or so until a full three months after surgery. If all continued to go well after that, she could return to four-to-six-month evaluations of her operated eye and the developing cataract in the left eye.

Complications

Although 96 to 98 percent of all cataract surgery is successful, it is worth considering what might happen in that 2 to 4 percent of cases where complications arise.

Postoperative Eye Infection

Postoperative eye infections are the first and most common complication. These range from a mild infection of the external eye tissues, such as the conjunctiva (which is cut during cataract surgery), to the far more serious intraocular (internal) infection. External infections are generally easily treated with antibiotic eyedrops or ointments. Internal infections can range from mild ones amenable to systemic antibiotic treatment to massive infections involving the entire eyeball and resulting in severe loss of vision.

Intraocular Inflammation

Intraocular inflammation is another common postoperative condition. This is not an infection (that is, it is not caused by foreign organisms such as bacteria or viruses). Rather, it is an inflammatory response to the trauma of the surgical procedure. This generally is minor and goes away by itself, but its resolution may be speeded with the use of cortisone or other steroid medications applied topically.

Hemorrhage

Hemorrhage is another possible postoperative complication. This, too, ranges from limited bleeding within the eye (usually the anterior chamber) that stops on its own and has no permanent effect to a massive hemorrhage with grave consequences. A very rare extreme is called an *expulsive choroidal hemorrhage.* The bleeding, generally from the choroid into the vitreous fluid, can occur during or after surgery and results in great visual loss or possible loss of the eye itself.

Secondary Glaucoma

Secondary glaucoma can result from cataract removal. Here, scar tissues or anatomical shifts caused by the surgery provoke an increase in the intraocular pressure. This can be mild and easily controlled with eyedrops, but in rare cases it can become severe, requiring corrective surgery. The iridectomy routinely performed as part of cataract surgery is a precaution against this complication.

A severe type of secondary glaucoma results when the normal flow of aqueous fluid from the anterior to posterior (forward to rear) chambers inside the eye is blocked by the vitreous fluid pressing up against the base of the iris. This condition, known as *pupillary block,* brings about a sudden rise in the pressure inside the eyeball. This is an emergency that necessitates a rapid surgical response.

Retinal Detachment

Although rare, *retinal detachment* is probably the most common potentially blinding complication of cataract surgery. Removing the posterior capsule increases the risk of retinal detachment, especially if an individual is very nearsighted or has *lattice degeneration,* a condition in which retinal tissue is thinned and its attachment weakened. For reasons not fully understood, retinal detachment occurs slightly more often in men than in women and also more often in younger people than in older people. A detached retina must be surgically corrected. This might be accomplished by heat or freezing in conjunction with conventional surgical means or by a laser beam.

Cystoid Macular Edema

Cystoid macular edema is swelling of the tissues of the macula, the most sensitive part of the retina. It is unclear what causes it, but it may be related to shifts in both pressure and the anatomical relationship within the eyeball. Whatever the cause, swelling in the highly vulnerable macula can cause visual distortion and even visual loss, depending on its severity. Medication or, very rarely, surgical intervention may be indicated to try to minimize this problem.

Flat Anterior Chamber

A flat anterior chamber is generally due to a slight leak in the surgical incision. A pressure bandage (tight gauze on the outside of the eye) often facilitates healing. If it does not in time heal on its own, the surgeon must correct it by reclosing the wound.

Postoperative Astigmatism

Postoperative astigmatism can be caused by sutures that are too tight and are pulling on the cornea in such a way that it is left distorted. The effect may be temporary or permanent, slight or pronounced. If necessary, this can be corrected with glasses or, most successfully, contact lenses.

Displacement of the Lens

Several complications are associated exclusively with lens implants. *Displacement of the lens* may be caused by trauma or may occur spontaneously. If the implant is dislocated, at best its optical advantage is eliminated and at worst it will cause health problems to the eye. Most commonly it is only partially dislocated, remaining in the visual axis and thus interfering with vision. In that case, it must be removed in a procedure that is, in essence, a second cataract extraction. Replacing it with a second implant is optional.

Secondary Cataracts

Secondary cataracts may develop when lens cells are not completely removed from the posterior capsule during extracapsular extraction. In one-quarter to one-half of cases, this tissue becomes clouded within five years after extracapsular surgery. Depending on the location of the newly opaque cells, the resultant visual impairment may be slight, requiring no treatment, or quite bothersome, necessitating further surgical correction to remove the offending lens remnants. That such postoperative complications will at times result in new secondary cataracts leads to the misunderstanding that a cataract can grow back after surgery.

A laser is usually used to burn a hole in the center of the opaque posterior capsule. When a hole is made into the posterior capsule, the protection that the posterior capsule gives against the complication of retinal detachment is eliminated. Hence one of the advantages of extracapsular surgery is eliminated when this complication arises.

If the lens remnant is too dense and hard to be cut by laser, the hole may have to be made mechanically with a knifelike instrument inserted into the eyeball. This is *discission* surgery. Again, keep in mind that the term secondary cataract does *not* refer to a cataract. It is a misnomer for a membrane left during cataract removal that has become opaque.

Cataract Surgery: Present and Future

In the early days of modern cataract surgery, 50 to 60 years ago, one of the most widely used procedures was extracapsular extraction without sutures. It is only in the last half century that suture material and needles fine enough and small enough for use in the eye have been available and in wide use. Before that, patients were confined to bed for up to two weeks with their heads immobilized between pillows and sandbags, to permit the wound to adhere and close on its own.

The popularity of the extracapsular technique as practiced earlier in this century can be attributed to the fact that a technique for intracapsular extraction, first performed in the late nineteenth century, had not yet evolved sufficiently to warrant its routine use. It was not until the 1930s and 1940s that the technique to remove the entire lens, nucleus, cortex, and anterior and posterior capsules as one came to predominate. Intracapsular extractions largely eliminated the complications associated with retained lens material.

The next big development was cryo-intracapsular cataract extraction, which is the most widely performed cataract procedure throughout the world today. In this variation a probe is used to freeze the entire lens into a single mass prior to extraction, thus making it easier to remove safely.

Sutures and needles became yet smaller and finer, and the tendency was to use a great many of them for better wound closure.

By the mid-1970s, cryo-intracapsular cataract extraction, still the safest technique known, promised a success rate of 98 percent. It is done mostly in the United States, where the much higher technology procedures are done, often at slightly higher risk.

In 1967 a procedure called *phakoemulsification* (literally, lens emulsification) was introduced. Here the lens is broken up inside the eye by vibration and the lens material is sucked out with an aspirating device. The posterior capsule is left in place. This procedure permits a far smaller incision to be made in the corneoscleral juncture (3 millimeters or so, in contrast to the standard 11-millimeter incision).

Phakoemulsification had an early burst of popularity, but that was interrupted by the advent of the lens implant. The implant requires a larger incision to get it into place, thus negating the main advantage of phakoemulsification. In recent years the procedure has regained some of its popularity, as smaller incisions can accommodate today's smaller implants. Phakoemulsification is used in about one-third of all cataract extractions performed today.

The most dramatic advance has been the intraocular (within the eye) lens implant. This was first tried experimentally in 1949 by Harold Ridley, a British ophthalmic surgeon who noticed that a World War II pilot had no rejection reaction to a piece of inert plastic from a Spitfire fighter plane lodged inside his eye. From this crude beginning, lens implants have been gradually improved and refined, with particular progress having been made over the last 15 years. They are now used in the vast majority of cataract operations in the United States.

Over the last ten years there has been a gradual return to extracapsular cataract extraction, surgical instruments and techniques having been improved immeasurably since these procedures were first developed. It is the surgical option of choice for lens implants because of the added stability to the implant as well as to the structures in the back of the eye. Today the majority of cataract extractions are extracapsular.

Solving the attendant problems of secondary cataracts is among the avenues of future progress that researchers are currently exploring. Scientists are looking for a nontoxic drug that will selectively destroy the remaining cortical or nuclear cells at the time of surgery to prevent opacification, while sparing the posterior capsule.

Newly available, but still being refined, are foldable lens implants. These afford the advantage of permitting smaller incisions, perhaps as small as 3 millimeters to 4 millimeters. Small incisions are theoretically better because they are less traumatic to the eye; all else being equal, the less the surgeon cuts, the better. Among refinements being developed is some means of chilling the lens in the folded position, making it technically easier to insert. The warmth of the eye would thaw the lens, which would unfold in place in the posterior chamber.

Smaller incisions are also paving the way for a single suture for closure. Special groovelike and ridgelike incisions may permit such good healing in a wound of 3 millimeters that eventually no suture at all might be required. A chemical or a little heat may be used to facilitate closure instead.

The theoretical advantages of using no sutures are that it entails less intervention and exposes the eye to fewer foreign bodies that can cause irritation or infection. In addition, postoperative astigmatism is less likely without sutures to pull on the wound as it heals. So the cycle may be nearing completion: from no sutures to a few, to many, and back to none; from extra- to intra-, and back to extracapsular extraction.

Bifocal and multifocal intraocular lens implants, although currently available, are in very limited use because of unsolved optical problems. Solutions to these problems are currently on the drawing board. Other types of intraocular lens implants under development are flexible lenses with ultraviolet absorption qualities. The UV absorption not only protects the retina but also results in more natural color vision, the lack of which some cataract patients are currently complaining about.

Laser phakoablation (a wearing away of the lens) is a surgical technique using laser technology. Still in the experimental stages, it would use fiberoptically guided laser beams to remove the cortex and nucleus, leaving a visually intact clear anterior and posterior capsule. This would then be filled with a new material whose refractive index would be very similar to that of the natural lens. These seeming fantasies today may become tomorrow's realities.

Another use for laser technology to look for in the future is *preventive laser scanning*. It is hoped that this technique can be used to detect the first traces of cataract formation by picking up protein changes in the lens and measuring their rate of growth. Combined with an experimental drug that may arrest or even reverse protein production, this technology holds the first theoretical promise for delaying cataract development to the point where surgery is not required for up to 20 years.

There is clearly an ever-brightening future for those who have cataracts, and the chances are that most of us will join that group at some point in our lives. As previously mentioned, over one million cataract operations are performed annually in the United States today, making it the most frequent operation on people over 65 years of age. It is true now, and will increasingly be so, that cataract surgery provides one of the most dramatic results obtainable in all of surgery. There is nothing more gratifying to a physician than restoring near-perfect vision to a patient facing eventual blindness.

About Glaucoma

◇

MYTH: Glaucoma is a cancer, a tumor, or an infection.
FACT: Glaucoma is none of these. It is a disease of the
eye in which pressure inside the eyeball is higher than it
should be. If left untreated, glaucoma can result in gradual
but permanent damage to sight.

MYTH: High blood pressure and the high eye pressure
of glaucoma are somehow related.
FACT: There is no connection whatever between elevated blood pressure and the increased eye pressure that
causes glaucoma. People with high blood pressure are not
more likely to develop glaucoma than people whose blood
pressure is normal, nor are glaucoma patients more prone
to high blood pressure.

Of all the possible causes of blindness, glaucoma is among
the most common, but it is also the easiest to prevent. If

undiagnosed and untreated, it will gradually cause loss of sight; if diagnosed early, glaucoma can be controlled and the loss of sight prevented. It is really as simple as that. What complicates matters is that in its most common form, glaucoma has no symptoms until extensive and irreversible damage has already been done, so that the only way you can obtain a positive early diagnosis is by visiting an ophthalmologist regularly.

Because glaucoma generally occurs after middle age, people over 40 should have periodic medical examinations of their eyes much more frequently than younger people should. Unlike cataracts, in which medical intervention is not necessary until the patient shows definite symptoms, treatment of glaucoma is most effective *before* the patient experiences symptoms. Especially if there is a history of glaucoma in your family, but even if there is none, yearly checkups by an ophthalmologist are a prudent course after you reach 40.

It is relatively simple for an eye doctor to spot glaucoma, and the rate of successful treatment is high. All the same, glaucoma is responsible each year for countless cases of blindness or extensive, permanent loss of vision. In the overwhelming majority of these cases, the damage could have been avoided. If all persons over 40 visited their eye doctor annually, glaucoma-induced blindness could be virtually eliminated.

What Is Glaucoma?

Glaucoma is an eye disease characterized by higher than normal pressure inside the eye (intraocular pressure). Pres-

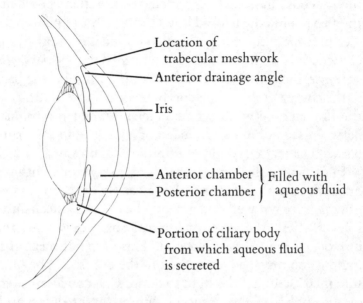

Fig. 7.1 **Where the aqueous fluid enters and drains from the eyeball**

sure can increase gradually or suddenly, slightly or dramatically, and for various reasons, depending on the type of glaucoma. By far the most common type is called *chronic simple glaucoma* (see page 153), in which the pressure increase is small, the beginning stages of the disease are without symptoms, and the progressive damage is slow and gradual. It occurs most commonly after age 40; in fact, about one out of 25 people past that age have chronic simple glaucoma.

To understand glaucoma it is important to understand what happens inside the eye when intraocular pressure increases. The inside surface of the cornea is nourished by the aqueous fluid, which is secreted by the ciliary body into the area behind the iris and flows through the pupil into the area in front of the iris. The aqueous fluid is reabsorbed and carried away to the blood at a point called the *anterior drainage angle,* located where the front of the iris joins the back of the cornea. It is here that problems arise. In a healthy eye the drainage network works efficiently, and the balance between secretion and drainage of aqueous fluid is maintained by a relatively constant intraocular pressure.

In glaucoma, however, something goes wrong with the drainage part of the process. For a variety of reasons, some of which are not well understood, the drainage mechanism is less efficient, the secretion/drainage balance is upset, and intraocular pressure is increased. This does not mean that there is too much aqueous fluid in the eye, since the pressure increase forces the fluid to drain. Glaucoma can affect one eye or both, but it is most common for it to affect both eyes.

Increased Intraocular Pressure

Increased intraocular pressure, even when it is very slight, tends to affect the human eye. The treatment for glaucoma is not designed to correct the underlying problem in the drainage mechanism; it aims instead to bring the pressure back down to normal. In this sense, glaucoma cannot be cured, but it can be controlled so that damage to the eye is avoided.

When intraocular pressure is too high, it causes damage to certain particularly delicate parts of the eye. We know that the eyeball has a very effective system of protective layers to prevent injury to its delicate internal structures. The sclera, which covers the entire eyeball except for the cornea and the place where the optic nerve enters the eye, is very tough, as is the cornea. The optic nerve, the vital connection between eye and brain, is not as tough, and it is vulnerable to elevated pressure. The increasing pressure affects the entire eye, making the eyeball harder than it should be and causing stress to all parts. The eye as a whole can withstand this without being damaged, but the delicate nerve fibers and blood vessels at the end of the optic nerve (the *optic disc*) cannot. If the pressure continues long enough, it will kill nerve fibers in the optic nerve, and once they have died they cannot be regenerated or replaced.

Glaucoma is referred to as a progressive disease, but it is really the damage it inflicts that is progressive. The defect in drainage does not necessarily get worse, nor does the pressure tend to increase steadily. But if untreated, the effect—killing off the cells of the optic nerve—continues, and the resulting loss of vision becomes progressively greater until the complete destruction of the optic nerve results in total blindness.

The nerve fibers at the outer edge of the optic disc are the first to go. In time, interior cells near the center die off. The outer edge corresponds to the outermost periphery of the retina and therefore to our outermost peripheral vision. Each succeeding layer of nerve fiber therefore corresponds to a more central area of the retina, and the innermost layers contain the nerve fibers that receive messages from the macula. As each layer dies, the peripheral visual field narrows, and finally central vision is lost. In the latter stages of untreated glaucoma, a person could have very narrow tunnel vision and be able to see nothing at all off to the sides but still have 20/20 vision when looking at objects

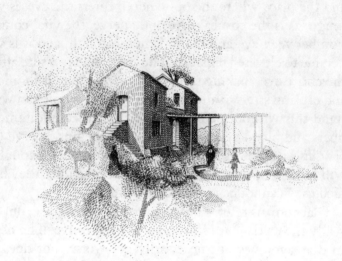

Fig. 7.2   Clear central vision (20/20) is received by the macula. Less-clear peripheral vision is received by the rest of the retina.

straight ahead. This is because it is the macula, and the macula only, that can deliver a 20/20 image to the brain.

People with untreated chronic glaucoma are rarely aware of the disease until a great deal of damage has already been done. The progressive death of nerve fibers takes place very slowly, and the elevation of pressure is usually too slight to cause pain or blurring of vision. Besides, we are all mostly unaware of what we see on the edges of our visual fields, because the messages received from that area of the retina are not very sharp and provide little more than our sense of the surrounding landscape. But even if the gradual loss of peripheral vision is imperceptible to us, it can be spotted when an ophthalmologist measures and diagrams the visual field.

Types of Glaucoma

Chronic Simple Glaucoma

The word *simple* in chronic simple glaucoma means that the pressure rise is not the result of any known underlying factor. Heredity seems to play some role but not a major one. This is why doctors test individuals with a family history of glaucoma even before they reach age 40. This does not mean everyone with a family history will develop the disease, or that it is impossible to find glaucoma in a person whose family has no history of it.

For reasons that are not well understood, people of African ancestry suffer glaucoma in significantly greater numbers than those of European ancestry. The greater pigmentation present in very dark eyes may be a contributing factor. In the United States, the incidence of glaucoma among African Americans is three times that of Caucasians.

The fact that chronic simple glaucoma often begins in the middle years does not explain the cause. Glaucoma is not like senile cataracts, which are part of the aging process and result from eye changes that always take place as we grow older. The closest we can come to an explanation is to say that glaucoma seems to develop in people who have a tendency toward inefficient drainage of aqueous fluid, and as these people grow older and their bodies as a whole lose their resiliency, the drainage problem reaches a point where it starts to cause problems.

Chronic simple glaucoma makes up about 95 percent of

all cases of glaucoma. There are other, rare types, which together make up the remaining 5 percent.

Chronic Secondary Glaucoma

This type has all the distinguishing features of chronic simple glaucoma except that the drainage defect is caused by something identifiable, most commonly a complication of another eye problem. Inflammation from an internal eye infection can be responsible for poor drainage; likewise, an allergic reaction within the eye, trauma, eye tumors, or scar tissue left by any of these problems can reduce drainage efficiency. Chronic secondary glaucoma can also be a complication of cataracts, because the diseased lens, which tends to be enlarged, can encroach upon the front of the eyeball and narrow or block the drainage angle. Medications such as corticosteroids can also be the cause, as can intraocular lens implants. Secondary glaucoma represents about 5 percent of all glaucoma cases.

Acute Glaucoma

Whether simple or secondary, acute glaucoma is a rare and dramatic condition (about one percent of all glaucomas can be classified as acute). The elevation of intraocular pressure becomes rapid and is many times higher than ever experienced with chronic glaucoma (60 and above for acute glaucoma, as compared to 20 to 25 for chronic glaucoma). The drainage angle is almost totally blocked, which causes the eyeball to become very hard. The pressure increase in chronic glaucoma is so slight that it can be detected only with special instruments, but the increased pressure in acute glaucoma can often be felt by merely touching the front of the eye with the fingers. The pressure is so great that it causes severe pain and damage to the whole eye. The cornea can become clouded, which results in blurred vision; blood vessels in the eyeball become swollen, causing pronounced redness; and the nerves surrounding the blood vessels respond to the pressure, causing great pain. Headaches, nausea, vomiting, and abdominal pains are symptoms that frequently accompany an acute glaucoma attack. The destructive effects on the optic nerve are equally rapid and severe, and immediate treatment and surgery are required.

Acute glaucoma can result when a drainage angle that has always been abnormally narrow suddenly becomes completely blocked; in this case it is called *acute simple glaucoma*. Or it can be a complication of a number of eye problems, including infection, allergic reaction, trauma, or cataracts. It is then called *acute secondary glaucoma*.

Congenital Glaucoma

This type of glaucoma is also quite rare (less than one percent of all glaucomas). It is present at birth or develops during infancy and is the result of an anatomical defect in which the drainage angle is very narrow or the drainage canals are malformed. It most commonly occurs in both eyes. The pressure elevation tends to be higher than in chronic glaucoma but not so extreme as in acute. The main characteristics of congenital glaucoma differ from the two other types, mostly because a baby's eyeball is much less tough than an adult's. The combination of the softer support tissues of an infant's eyeball and the considerably increased intraocular pressure cause significant enlargement of the eyeball. Therefore, children with congenital glaucoma can often be recognized by their disproportionately large eyes. Surgery is usually necessary, and it must be performed early if permanent loss of sight is to be avoided.

Low-Tension Glaucoma

This type of glaucoma is very rare, occurring in fewer than one percent of all cases of glaucoma. As the name suggests, the eye exhibits signs of glaucoma damage even though the pressure is within the normal range. The explanation is that the affected eye requires a lower-than-normal eye pressure to avoid damage to the optic nerve, so pressure levels that would be normal for other eyes are exerting stresses in that eye.

Low-tension glaucoma is more difficult to diagnose early than chronic simple glaucoma because the clue, increased intraocular pressure, is absent. This glaucoma is virtually always diagnosed after damage to the visual field and optic disc has occurred. An ophthalmologist may see signs of the damage during a routine exam, or a visual field test done for another reason may reveal characteristic narrowing of peripheral vision. Occasionally, the glaucoma is advanced far enough to cause visual symptoms that bring an individual to an ophthalmologist. The symptoms include bumping into objects because of a severely constricted peripheral visual field.

Low-tension glaucoma should not be confused with low eye pressure. A severe perforating injury to the eye may cause aqueous and, possibly, vitreous fluid to drain from the eye, which will bring about severely low eye pressure. This is analogous to low blood pressure when a person goes into shock, and it is an emergency situation. This is still the only time when low eye pressure is a medical problem. And, of course, intraocular pressure has nothing to do with blood pressure.

How Glaucoma Is Diagnosed

Intraocular pressure that is below 20 or 25 (depending on the instrument used to measure it) is generally considered normal. There is a certain amount of variation, however, since pressure will change constantly as the natural balance of aqueous secretions and drainage differs during the course of the day. Pressure may be higher (or lower) in the morning than in the afternoon, or higher one day than the next. Furthermore, the amount of pressure a given eye can withstand without damage also varies, so what is elevated pressure for one person might not be a medical problem for another.

Because glaucoma is quite rare under age 40, pressure readings are not necessarily part of the routine eye examination before that age, unless there is a family history or the ophthalmologist spots an abnormality during the routine exam that warrants measuring the pressure. Some ophthalmologists, however, might take a baseline pressure reading the first time they see a patient, regardless of age. After age 40 a pressure reading is a routine part of the annual eye exam. If the results are normal, it is safe to let a year elapse before testing again.

Routine Testing

Pressure is tested with an instrument called a *tonometer*. The two basic types of tests are *Schiotz tonometry* and *applanation tonometry.* Both are done after anesthetic drops are put in the eye. These allow the ophthalmologist to touch the instrument to the eyeball without causing discomfort. The effect wears off within about 20 minutes.

The Tonometer

The Schiotz tonometer is held by the ophthalmologist while the patient is tilted back in the examining chair. The applanation tonometer, the most frequently used, allows the patient to sit upright at the biomicroscope, to which the tonometer is attached. It is used with an orange dye that is visible in blue light emitted by the biomicroscope. A third

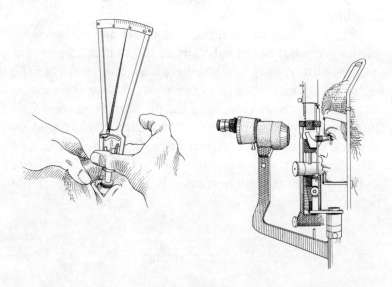

Fig. 7.3   Two ways to test for glaucoma, Schiotz (left) and applanation (right) tonometers

type, which is slightly less accurate, involves no contact with the eyeball and, therefore, requires no anesthetic drops. Called *noncontact applanation,* it employs a controlled air pulse, which the patient feels as a brief cool blast of air on the eye. This method may be helpful if a patient has an external infection, making it inadvisable to physically touch the cornea.

Ophthalmologists routinely examine the front anatomy of the eye and the optic disc of all patients regardless of age. In patients over 40, the doctor will be looking for specific signs that may suggest glaucoma.

The front anatomy is viewed with the biomicroscope through an undilated pupil to give the ophthalmologist a sense of the depth of the anterior chamber—whether it looks normal, shallow, or quite deep. If it is shallow, drainage may be less efficient than in a normal or deep chamber.

Viewing the Optic Disc

Evaluating the health of the optic nerve is of particular importance in diagnosing and managing glaucoma because this is where most of the damage to the eye, and to one's vision, occurs. What the doctor looks for in the optic disc is a condition called *cupping.* A normal optic disc is basically level with the retina and should appear pinkish-yellow in color. As glaucoma progresses, the increasingly damaged disc begins to show an indentation. The more severe this indentation, the greater the damage, and it also becomes paler and more yellow as the disease interferes with blood circulation to the optic disc.

Three methods are available for viewing the optic disc, all of which require the pupils to be dilated. The most common is direct ophthalmoscopy: The examiner uses a hand-held ophthalmoscope and very bright light. Standing very close to the patient, he or she peers into the pupil for an illuminated view of the optic disc. Indirect ophthalmoscopy employs a bright light that the ophthalmologist wears strapped to the head like a miner's lamp. Holding a large lens in front of the eye and standing a foot or so from the patient, the examiner shines the light through the lens into the eye. A third method uses the biomicroscope and what is called a *Hruby lens,* which gives a three-dimensional view of the disc to clearly show any cupping.

The final routine test is an evaluation of the patient's visual field, in which the ophthalmologist wiggles a pencil or other object out to the sides while the patient looks straight ahead. This will give the doctor an idea if a more extensive and precise field test is warranted. Some ophthalmologists may do a full-blown visual field test on their older patients, even when no suggestive findings turn up in the routine exam. The test is given just to get a baseline record of the field.

If the results of all of these tests are normal, no further evaluations are needed for a year. Additional testing must be done, however, if pressure is above 20 (measured with Schiotz tonometry) or 25 (with applanation tonometry), or if there is evidence of abnormality in the anatomy of the anterior chamber, damage to the optic nerve, or narrowing of the visual field.

Specialized Glaucoma Testing

The ophthalmologist will schedule a second appointment for other tests if necessary. One reason is that these tests are time-consuming, and most patients prefer to be prepared in advance if they must spend considerable additional time at the doctor's office. Another reason is that some people may need to prepare themselves psychologically for the battery of tests, which are ordered because the doctor suspects a serious eye disease. Finally, because the progression of tests requires tonometry to be done at the end of the initial exam, after the eyes are dilated, and this might influence the pressure reading, a confirming pressure reading should be done on undilated eyes.

Intraocular pressure is not static, and dilation is just one of the factors that might cause a variation in pressure readings. Because it changes over the course of the day and from day to day, some doctors might schedule the second examination for a different time of day in order to pinpoint any such variations.

There is a series of tests that, taken together, will confirm the diagnosis of glaucoma. If at some point in the course of the tests the ophthalmologist is certain the patient has glaucoma, the full series of tests may not be done. The time and expense are not justified if a definitive diagnosis can be made on the basis of fewer tests. Nonetheless, some tests or examination procedures are always part of a glaucoma evaluation. Even if glaucoma is diagnosed, the tests are repeated regularly as part of glaucoma management.

Gonioscopy

After rechecking the intraocular pressure in each eye, the ophthalmologist examines the drainage angle with a specially designed contact lens called a *gonioscope*. It has mirrors and facets to give an illuminated view of a normally dark corner of the eye that is at a 90-degree angle from the examiner. Inserted painlessly into the anesthetized eye and

used in conjunction with the biomicroscope, the gonioscope allows a close-up view of the angle where aqueous
fluid flows into the drainage canal. The gonioscope is
inserted into each eye to determine if the drainage angle in
either eye appears anatomically normal, open but somewhat inadequate, or narrowed. This examination is always
included in a diagnostic series and if the patient has glaucoma, it may be repeated periodically to monitor changes
in the drainage angle.

Stress Test

Stressing the drainage mechanism by giving it extra fluid to
drain through an angle that is narrowed by dilation will
tend to increase intraocular pressure. This may help determine if a borderline pressure reading is normal for that
patient or if it is clearly a sign of glaucoma. A slight increase
in intraocular tension on a stress test is normal; an increase
of over 5 or 6 is considered abnormal.

The patient drinks about a liter (slightly less than a quart)
of water over the course of about five minutes, then sits in
a dark room for about 30 minutes. The pressure is measured
with a tonometer and compared with the reading taken at
the beginning of the evaluation.

The idea here is that the water somewhat increases the
secretion of aqueous fluid into the eyes, adding stress to the
outflow mechanism. The dark room dilates the pupils, anatomically narrowing the drainage angles and adding further stress to the aqueous fluid outflow. Although this is an
artificial situation, it tends to reveal any slight tendency for
poor drainage.

The stress test is not always performed. For example,
when pressure readings are high enough to leave no doubt

that an individual has glaucoma, a stress test is not necessary. Sometimes it is done as an adjunct to tonography.

Tonography

The test of *tonography,* which is not used very frequently, estimates how efficiently aqueous fluid flows out from the anterior chamber. It relies on the phenomenon that massaging an eye tends to lower its intraocular pressure temporarily by speeding drainage from the anterior chamber. The effect is marked in normal eyes, but occurs at a slower rate in glaucomatous eyes.

Using an instrument to massage the eyes, then measuring the drop in pressure as the aqueous fluid drains gives the ophthalmologist a picture of drainage efficiency. With the eyes anesthetized and the patient lying on an examining table, an electronic Schiotz-type tonometer is applied to the cornea for about four minutes. The tonometer produces a massage effect and thereby expresses the fluid from the anterior chamber. The changes in pressure over the four-minute period are printed out on a strip of graph paper.

It is important to note that even though the very slight external pressure on the eyeball for this brief test will in no way damage either a healthy or glaucomatous eye, eye massage should not be considered a therapeutic approach in glaucoma. Nor should one try to prevent the development of glaucoma with eye massage.

Tonography is not always included as part of the standard glaucoma evaluation. When it is, it may be repeated as a stress test: Following the stress test already described, the ophthalmologist takes the four-minute tonographic reading again.

Visual Field Tests

The next step in every glaucoma diagnostic evaluation is examination of the visual field. There are numerous types of visual field tests. All yield a sort of map consisting of: the area of central vision (the macula), where vision is most acute and where smaller and weaker visual stimuli can be perceived; peripheral vision, where increasingly larger and stronger stimuli are needed to get a test response; and finally, the normal blind spot of the eye, where no stimuli are seen, regardless of size or intensity.

Damage to the optic nerve is reflected as narrowing of the visual field, from the outer edges inward, and an enlargement of the blind spot. Increased cupping of the optic disc tends to occur at the same rate as visual field constriction, and in this sense these findings confirm one another.

Because mapping the visual field is important in keeping track of the progression of glaucoma, it is more than a diagnostic tool. It is repeated periodically (usually every six months) as part of glaucoma management.

The *tangent screen* (see Figure 7.4) is a large blackboard-like screen that hangs on a wall. The patient sits one meter in front of the screen and the visual field of each eye is charted separately, with the other eye covered. In a dimly illuminated room, the patient stares straight ahead at a brightly lit white dot in the center of the screen while the examiner brings in objects to be viewed at various sizes from the side, and from above and below. The patient tells the examiner when the test object first becomes visible. The examiner places map pins on the tangent screen at points corresponding to the areas the patient indicates. In this way the shape and size of the visual field are outlined, including

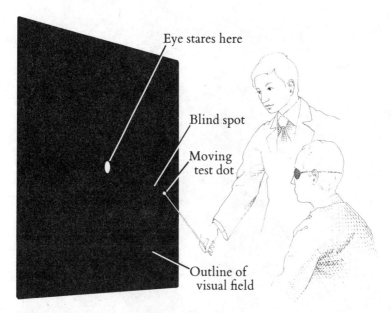

Fig. 7.4 The tangent screen

the shape and size of the blind spot. When the test is completed for one eye, the procedure is repeated for the other eye. This type of visual field test is not frequently used today.

Electronic field testers are a more modern development that give a slightly faster result and are easier for a technician to use than the tangent screen. The one most frequently used is called a *perimeter*. In a dimly lit room, the patient sits in front of a half-globelike device (see Figure 7.5). One eye is covered, and the chin sits on a chin rest. The patient is instructed to keep the uncovered eye fixed straight ahead at all times. A telescope-like device in the middle of the globe permits the examiner to center the eye.

The patient is presented with visual stimuli, dots of light

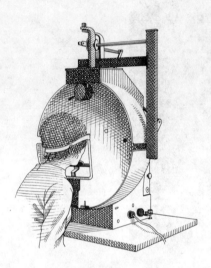

Fig. 7.5   **Testing visual fields with the perimeter.**

in various sizes and intensities, and at various locations throughout the inside surface of the half globe. He or she is instructed to ring a buzzer whenever a dot of light becomes visible. The buzzer signal avoids the need to talk, which would cause head movement and thus alter the patient's constant straight-ahead position. As with the tangent screen, the patient's responses permit the examiner to plot out the visual field.

Static perimetry employs a series of electronically produced test stimuli (blips of light), but instead of moving around a screen, each is in a fixed position. The stimulus is initially too dim to be seen, but is gradually brightened until the patient indicates that it is visible. This is repeated until the borders of the visual field are established. This method is more time-consuming.

Automated perimeters are computer-driven visual field testers, which are a great advantage when trained ophthalmic personnel are not available. These machines produce a printout of the visual field based on patient responses processed by the computer rather than recorded by a trained examiner.

On the other end of the technological spectrum is a portable visual field test called *oculo-kinetic perimetry*. It is useful for bedridden or housebound patients, or in developing countries where the machine must go to the patient. The test is done with a test chart, record sheet, and pencil, and differs from the others in that the patient's eye, rather than the test stimuli, is what moves. This simple and economical test yields somewhat less complete and accurate data, but it is of value when portability is a factor.

Fundus Photography

Although not strictly speaking a glaucoma test, special 3-D photographs can be taken of the optic disc. Known as fundus photography, it can be used to compile a visual record of the state of the optic disc at the time of each examination. The photographs permit the ophthalmologist to track damage to the optic disc, comparing earlier and later photographs. Some ophthalmologists have photographs taken at the time of diagnosis; others may wait until the patient is under treatment. Some ophthalmologists have the specialized equipment required to take the photographs in their office; others will refer the patient to an eye clinic at a local hospital, much as one might do for X rays or other high-tech imaging.

What the Tests Mean

With the information gained from the gonioscopy, tonometric or possibly tonographic tests, ophthalmoscopic
examination of the optic disc, and charting of the visual
fields, an ophthalmologist can make a diagnosis. There are
three possibilities: First, the tests may reveal no abnormalities, suggesting that the elevated reading was an exception.
The patient would then be told he or she does not have
glaucoma and will be asked simply to return in one year for
the routine checks as part of the annual eye exam. Second,
if the pressure readings or tests (or both) are borderline, the
patient joins what is referred to as a *glaucoma-suspect* group,
meaning no treatment is required but the situation should
be monitored with reevaluations every six months. Such an
individual is clearly at increased risk for developing glaucoma. Finally, the tests might be unequivocally abnormal,
leading to the diagnosis of glaucoma.

A Rare Emergency

A pressure over 40 might indicate acute glaucoma or severe
chronic glaucoma. In this unusual circumstance, the doctor
will do confirming tests and institute treatment immediately to avoid further damage to the eye. Examinations
include a visual field test and gonioscopy. The optic disc
will also be looked at; if the pupils have not already been
dilated, the ophthalmologist will do the exam without
dilating them, since this might aggravate the pressure elevation. Tonography would probably not be performed, and
stress testing would obviously be contraindicated.

With more severe glaucoma, treatment efforts would be

made to reduce the pressure immediately and quickly. This might be done by instilling drops to constrict the pupil (mechanically widening the drainage angle) every 15 to 30 minutes while pressure is monitored. Pressure could also be reduced by diuretic pills or injected pressure-lowering medication.

In acute glaucoma, laser surgery will probably be required to improve the anatomical condition that contributed to the sudden and severe rise in pressure.

8

If You Have Glaucoma

◇

MYTH: You will be able to tell if you have glaucoma because you will experience eye pain, see halos around lights, have excessive tearing, or your eyes will bother you in some other way.

FACT: Although there is a rare form of glaucoma that can be quite painful, the most common type causes no pain at all and is without symptoms until the disease is far advanced.

MYTH: You should not drink liquids, especially coffee and alcohol, if you have glaucoma.

FACT: This notion is a holdover from years ago, when glaucoma patients were advised to reduce their intake of liquids. Modern treatment methods make this unnecessary. A glaucoma patient today can lead a perfectly normal life as long as the prescribed medication is taken as directed.

MYTH: If you have glaucoma, you will feel pressure in your eyes.
FACT: Increased intraocular pressure, unless very high, causes no symptoms, so patients with chronic simple glaucoma do not feel increased pressure in their eyes.

MYTH: When glaucoma is diagnosed and treated, its damage can be corrected.
FACT: The damage to the eye that has already occurred cannot be undone. That is why it is so important to detect glaucoma early.

If you have chronic simple glaucoma, by far the most common of all glaucoma types, the chances are you will first learn of it from an eye doctor, who will have seen signs of it in the course of a routine medical eye examination. Because chronic simple glaucoma is completely without symptoms—no pain, no discernible visual loss—until its later stages, the annual visit to an ophthalmologist is of enormous importance. This is particularly true after age 40, when glaucoma is most likely to occur.

Because of the seriousness of glaucoma, some people mistakenly believe that visits to an optometrist to have glasses or contact lenses fitted are a reasonable substitute for regular examinations by an ophthalmologist. Many optometrists routinely do a preliminary screening test for ocular pressure, especially for older patients. If you find yourself at an optometrist's office and he or she doesn't perform such a test, ask for it. If the results are even borderline, the optometrist should recommend that you make an appointment with an ophthalmologist promptly. However, it is best to see an ophthalmologist regularly.

If you are diagnosed as having glaucoma, your experience will likely be similar to that of the patient described below.

The First Visit

Mr. B was 49 years old when he came in for his annual ophthalmological examination. His only complaint was that the reading glasses prescribed for him three years before now seemed too weak. In the course of the examination, his doctor found that he did indeed require stronger reading glasses, a normal finding considering his age.

Because Mr. B is over 40, his intraocular pressure was tested as a matter of course. On this visit, the readings by applanation tonometry were somewhat elevated at 28 in the right eye, and at 25, which is borderline, in the left eye.

Routine examination of the front anatomy of each eye under the biomicroscope and of each optic disc with the ophthalmoscope showed findings that were all within normal limits. The gross visual field test done by moving a test object around the periphery of his vision was also normal. In addition to these tests, which pertain specifically to glaucoma, the ophthalmologist performed a full medical eye examination, and all findings were within normal limits.

Mr. B's ophthalmologist told him that, except for the test of his intraocular pressure, the examination was normal. But because pressure elevation could be an indication of early glaucoma, it must be investigated further. Intraocular pressure changes constantly as the dynamic secretion and drainage of aqueous fluid changes, from hour to hour and day to day. A single abnormal pressure reading would not automatically point to glaucoma, and more extensive tests would be needed.

There were three possibilities: First, subsequent pressure readings and special tests would not reveal any significant abnormalities, from which it could be concluded that Mr. B did not have glaucoma and would simply be rechecked as usual in one year. In that case, the single high pressure reading would probably have been the result of normal fluctuation. Second, the pressures and some or all of the tests would be borderline, which would put him into the glaucoma-suspect group. In that case, no treatment would be instituted, but he would be reevaluated on a six-month basis because he was clearly at increased risk for developing glaucoma. The third possibility—that pressures and/or tests were abnormal—would mean that he had glaucoma. He would need treatment, probably in the form of eye drops, which would control, but not cure, the disease and would have to be used for the rest of his life.

The Second Visit

Mr. B returned a week later, prepared to spend several hours in the doctor's office. The first part of the glaucoma evaluation was done without dilating his eyes. Instead, the doctor used anesthetic drops, which took immediate effect and kept his eyes numb for about 20 minutes. This time the applanation tonometer revealed pressures of 30 and 26 in his right and left eyes, respectively. Pressure in the right eye was slightly more elevated than on the initial exam, and the left eye was again borderline.

Gonioscopic examination of the anterior chamber of the right eye and its drainage angle showed an open angle but also revealed some abnormal fibrous tissue and some increased pigmentation in the *trabecular meshwork,* the tissue through which the aqueous fluid drains from the eye. The left eye had an open angle and very minimally abnormal fibrous tissue, with no increase in pigmentation in the trabecular area.

Because of the borderline reading on the left eye, and to confirm the reading on the right, the ophthalmologist decided to do tonography and stress testing.

The first tonographic reading was taken for four minutes while Mr. B lay on his back. He was then given nearly a quart of water to drink, and the room was darkened. After about a half hour, more anesthetic drops were instilled before a tonometric reading was taken and the tonography repeated.

The stress test indicated an abnormal pressure rise in the right eye, and a rise in the left eye that was within normal limits. Mr. B's right eye, unlike a normal eye, could not adequately absorb the stress of added fluid and anatomical narrowing.

Because the ophthalmologist observed no changes in the optic disc upon examining it with the ophthalmoscope during the annual visit, it was decided that fundus photographs would not be taken at this time. Should there begin to be changes at a later date, keeping a photographic record would be desirable.

Mr. B's doctor used the perimeter to map the visual field, a process that takes 15 to 20 minutes.

The visual fields were normal in both eyes, confirming the observation that the optic discs showed no signs of damage.

The doctor decided the left eye needed no treatment at this time but should be monitored closely because repeated borderline tensions place it in the "glaucoma-suspect category," the term used by ophthalmologists. Given the increased pressure in the right eye, anatomical abnormalities (scar tissue and increased pigmentation), and the abnormal stress test, the doctor decided to treat the right eye.

Mr. B is now given the good news that the examination shows no damage to his eyes. Nonetheless, he does have glaucoma in the right eye, and the left warrants follow-up as a so-called glaucoma-suspect eye.

Although a few ophthalmologists believe that glaucoma should not be treated until the first signs of definitive damage appear, Mr. B's doctor preferred to avoid any damage by prescribing one of the mildest eyedrops available. This would help establish and maintain normal intraocular pressure.

The doctor asked the patient to use the drops twice a day in the right eye. Mr. B would not have to alter his life-style or habits in any other way: He could read all he wanted, watch movies or TV as much as he liked, and eat or drink whatever he wished.

He was instructed to return in a week. Once the doctor was satisfied with his eye pressure, Mr. B would need to return every three months for monitoring of both eyes. This would involve pressure checks and, at six-month intervals, a visual field examination. The other specialized tests might be repeated periodically as needed. And, of course, Mr. B would need to continue coming in for his regular annual complete eye examinations.

The doctor explained that glaucoma cannot be cured, but it could be controlled, usually without too much difficulty. Also, the chances were good that Mr. B would never be bothered by it in any practical way, other than having to remember to take the medication.

One Week Later

When Mr. B returned a week later, his intraocular pressure was within normal limits in the treated right eye and unchanged in the left. He complained that the drops burned a bit, and that for the first two or three days he had a slight pulling sensation across his brow and some slightly funny visual effects. His doctor explained that the preservatives in the eyedrops might make them burn a bit. The pulling sensation and blurring (caused by slight and transient myopia) are not uncommon when these drops are first taken or changed. The doctor reassured Mr. B that the drops were doing their job and that the annoying side effects would soon pass. He was instructed to continue with the twice-a-day regimen and return in three months, unless the symptoms from the drops lasted more than two weeks. In that case, Mr. B should call the doctor's office.

Three Months Later

At this visit, Mr. B's vision was checked, pressure readings were taken in both eyes, and the eyes were examined under the biomicroscope and with the ophthalmoscope. Everything was satisfactory and unchanged. Mr. B was advised to continue using the eyedrops as he had.

Mr. B asked what would happen if his pressure went up while on these drops. His doctor explained that the drops he was using were quite weak, the mildest form available that could effectively control his eye pressure. If his pressure increased while on the drops, a checkup every three months would ensure that an elevation would be spotted before it did any damage. If such an elevation should occur, the doctor would prescribe one of the numerous stronger eyedrops available, or add a second drop to the regimen. If none of these succeeded in keeping the pressure down, pills could be prescribed to control intraocular pressure.

Concerned that three months is too long an interval between visits, Mr. B asked if there was a test he could do at home to keep closer tabs on his intraocular pressure. His doctor reassured him that, in a reasonably controlled situation such as his, three months was a safe interval and that there was no home test.

Prescribing glaucoma medication is done in steps, using the mildest possible formulation and keeping a close watch for changes. As is true in the practice of medicine in general, it is most desirable to use the smallest dose of the weakest drug that will do the job.

Six Months After the Diagnosis

Mr. B returned again three months later. His doctor examined his eyes and vision, and tested his pressure. In addition, his visual field was charted to ensure that no visual loss had occurred. Again, all was stable. He was advised to continue with the eyedrops and to return in three more months.

Three Years After the Diagnosis

Monitoring continued on a three-month basis. When Mr. B came in for his examination three years after the initial diagnosis, the first signs of change were noted in the previously untreated, but glaucoma-suspect, left eye. Pressure was elevated, and the fibrous tissue in the drainage angle had increased to an abnormal level. As confirmation, the ophthalmologist asked Mr. B to return two days later to have his pressure reading rechecked. The results were again the same.

The doctor prescribed the same drops as Mr. B had been using in his right eye, so he would now put them in both eyes twice a day. When he returned a week later, the pressure in the left eye was under control, and he was allowed to return to his three-month examination schedule.

Two-and-a-half Years Later

All continued normally for two-and-a-half years, until the doctor noted a slight increase in the pressure in the right eye. For the first time, a minimal suggestion of early cupping of the right optic disc was evident on ophthalmoscopic examination. This was accompanied by minimal early changes in his visual field. In response to this, the doctor prescribed a new eyedrop in addition to the one Mr. B had been using in both eyes. The new drop would be used in the right eye only.

In order to document changes in the optic disc, the doctor ordered fundus photographs. The fundus photos showed the early cup in the right eye and a normal disc in the left.

To confirm that the added drops were working, Mr. B was asked to return in a week for tonometry, and indeed things were again stabilized.

The Next Decade

Mr. B's condition was unchanged for the next three years. The doctor noted another pressure increase in the right eye and further cupping of the right optic disc as compared to the fundus photographs taken three years earlier. The doctor discontinued the two kinds of drops for the right eye, replacing them with a stronger formulation to be instilled four times a day instead of two. The left eye continued to get the single mild drop twice a day. Reexamination a week later showed Mr. B's intraocular pressure under control.

The three-month visits continued, with visual field examinations every other visit. There were no discernible changes for the next four years and six months, at which time changes again showed up in the right visual field, accompanied by an increase in pressure. The left eye continued to be stable on medication.

It is important to note that Mr. B was completely unaware of the changes in the visual field detected by the ophthalmologist. They were subtle and did not interfere with his acute central vision. This silent, symptomless feature of glaucoma is what makes close monitoring of all glaucoma patients so important. A medical checkup every three months and twice-yearly visual field testing will alert the physician that the disease is not under control and that the treatment regimen needs to be modified to restore normal pressure.

Mr. B received a new prescription: still stronger eyedrops four times a day in the right eye. The left eye was treated as before. Recheck a week later showed an improvement in the pressure but it was still a bit high, so a second drop was added. This controlled the pressure.

A year and nine months later, the left eye showed an increase in pressure and, on gonioscopy, increased narrowing and pigmentation. A second drop twice a day was prescribed to supplement the drops Mr. B had been using for nearly 12 years. On recheck, the ophthalmologist found that this controlled the left eye pressure.

Three years later, or some 18 years after the initial diagnosis, Mr. B was 67 years old. He was using several different eyedrops: one drop four times daily and a second one two times daily in his right eye; and two different drops, each used two times daily, in the left. He had had some visual field loss in the right eye, still none in the left. His central corrected vision continued to be 20/20 in both eyes.

From a practical point of view, Mr. B had noticed no visual deterioration in the 18 years since his glaucoma was diagnosed. He was annoyed by the need to use so many eyedrops several times a day, and he felt anxious before each of his three-month checkups. All in all, however, he acknowledged that it had been a small price to pay for continued normal vision and the chance that it would continue long into the future.

Glaucoma Therapy

As is evident from Mr. B's case, long-term glaucoma treatment can be accomplished with medications in the form of eyedrops. This is the first and most common approach to controlling intraocular pressure. If eyedrops do not work, medication taken orally or by another means can either replace or be added to the drops. Finally, surgery is available when all else fails.

Eyedrops

Eyedrops have been used to treat glaucoma for more than a century, and new glaucoma medications are being developed all the time. The earliest medication, pilocarpine, is derived from the leaves or roots of a South American shrub. It is classed as a miotic, which means it constricts the pupil of the eye. When the iris closes down around the pupil, it is drawn away from the drainage angle in the anterior chamber. This will mechanically widen the angle and facilitate aqueous outflow.

Other glaucoma medications act by decreasing the secretion of aqueous fluid, thus lowering pressure by reducing the amount of fluid to be drained. Timolol maleate (most frequently prescribed as Timoptic), the most widely used eyedrop for glaucoma, acts in this way. This and some other antiglaucoma drops may work also by exerting a pull on the trabecular meshwork, the net of fibers in the drainage angle. The effect is to increase aqueous fluid outflow at the site.

One or more different drops can be used in combination, either to enhance the effect on a single mechanism (aqueous production or drainage, or pupil constriction) or to affect different mechanisms. Some drops contain ingredients that produce a combination of effects. One of these is dipivefrin (most often prescribed as Propine), which slightly decreases aqueous production at the same time it increases the facility of outflow. It may be effectively used in conjunction with a pupil-constricting drop.

In any case, the weakest concentration used the least number of times daily is the first to be tried, with stronger drops prescribed and greater frequency added only if and when necessary to control pressure.

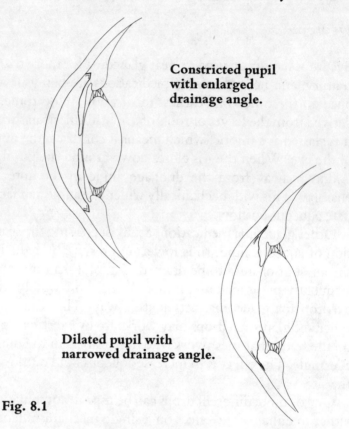

Constricted pupil
with enlarged
drainage angle.

Dilated pupil with
narrowed drainage angle.

Fig. 8.1

To help avoid confusion for patients who may be taking several different drops in combination, many are packaged with color-coded tops.

Some of the more common side effects of antiglaucoma drops include burning and redness, especially when they are used for the first time. Most eye medications contain preservatives to keep them sterile, and it is the preservative that is usually responsible for the irritation and stinging sensation. Some drops are available in single-dose ampules

tingling of the fingers and toes, and sometimes a distur-
bance in the body's chemical balance.

Intravenous Medication

When necessary, there are injectable drugs available to rapidly decrease intraocular pressure. These are primarily used
for acute glaucoma or to prepare an eye for intraocular surgery, when lower than normal pressure is an advantage.
These medications are hyperosmotic drugs; they act by
thickening the blood, which draws the thinner aqueous
fluid from the eye by a natural process called osmosis,
thereby reducing eye pressure. They work rapidly because
they do not depend on the normal drainage channels to
remove the aqueous; rather, the fluid is taken up by the tiny
blood vessels throughout the anterior chamber.

Glaucoma Surgery

In the overwhelming majority of cases, glaucoma can be
safely and effectively treated with medication. In the rare
cases when it cannot, surgical means are available. Unlike
cataract surgery, however, glaucoma surgery is not cura-
tive. Instead, it is another means to control the pressure ele-
vations, and it is usually necessary to continue drug therapy.
It is also often necessary to repeat the surgical procedures in
the future.

If you need surgery to relieve your glaucoma, your experience is likely to be similar to that of the patients described
here.

Ms. C was 51 years old when she saw an ophthalmologist for the first time in her life. She had a bad case of acute conjunctivitis in both eyes, with severe swelling, discharge, and discomfort. She had never had problems with her eyes before and never needed glasses when she was a young woman. When presbyopia forced her to get reading glasses, she bought them from a discount optical chain whose optician checked her vision but did not examine her eyes medically.

The ophthalmologist treated the conjunctivitis with antibiotic ointment and drops, and within two weeks the infection was completely cured. At that time the ophthalmologist did a complete medical eye examination. The reading of intraocular pressure, which was included as a matter of routine for anyone Ms. C's age, revealed 29 applanation in the left eye and 27 applanation in the right. She was instructed to return for a complete glaucoma evaluation.

On that visit the tensions were 31 left, 27 right. The increase in the left eye pressure might represent a typical day-to-day variation. Gonioscopy indicated that fibrous tissue in the drainage angles of both eyes, though worse in the left, was clearly interfering with normal aqueous outflow.

Visual field studies showed moderately advanced, irreversible changes in the left eye, including considerable enlargement of the blind spot and constriction in the peripheral vision. The right eye showed early though again irreversible changes: a slight blind spot enlargement with no peripheral constriction.

The ophthalmologist judged that stress and tonography tests would serve no purpose because it was already clear from his findings that Ms. C had glaucoma in both eyes. However, he took stereoscopic fundus photographs to have a documentary record of both optic discs.

The doctor told Ms. C that she definitely had glaucoma in both eyes and had sustained irreversible damage to her visual field. Thanks to the eye infection that brought her to an ophthalmologist for a medical checkup, treatment to control the glaucoma could begin before the disease did further damage. The doctor assured her that the eye infection in no way contributed to the glaucoma and that in all likelihood medications would keep the disease from worsening or at least slow it so significantly that she would retain useful vision for the rest of her life.

Ms. C was immediately placed on antiglaucoma drops, which initially decreased her pressure but controlled it adequately for only six months. Noting that her pressure was again elevated, the doctor prescribed a second eyedrop and gradually increased its strength and frequency over the next four visits.

This reasonably controlled events for about a year. Although the visual field change continued to be minimal in the right eye, there was some progression in the left. The doctor added oral medication to the regimen, and things were kept in check for about 18 months, after which the pressure in the left eye was again too high. Its visual field showed continued loss, and there was also further enlargement of the blind spot. Repeat fundus photos were taken and compared to the initial ones. Further cupping of the left optic disc confirmed the findings of the visual field test.

Because Ms. C was taking the greatest amount of the strongest medications available, the next step was surgery on the left eye. Surgery was not needed on the right eye: Pressure was within normal limits and its visual field was stable because of medical therapy.

Laser surgery was suggested because it is an essentially painless procedure, can be done on an outpatient basis in the

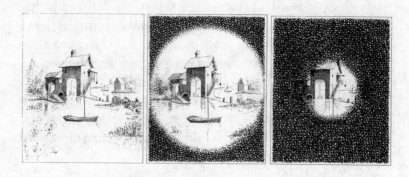

Fig. 8.2 Uncontrolled glaucoma can result in progressive narrowing of the field of vision: *(left)* controlled glaucoma, with no visual loss; *(center)* uncontrolled glaucoma, with some loss of peripheral vision; *(right)* advanced uncontrolled glaucoma, with serious loss of peripheral vision.

hospital eye clinic, and most important, is the safest surgical choice. Because this was not an emergency, the ophthalmologist told Ms. C she should feel free to seek a second opinion. Although often not required by health insurers in the case of laser eye surgery, getting a second opinion is a particularly wise precaution because laser procedures on the eyes are among the most unnecessary and widely overused surgical procedures in the United States today. It cannot be stressed too strongly that if you are advised to get laser eye surgery, get a second opinion.

Another ophthalmologist confirmed that surgery was

indicated, and her personal physician told her there was no medical reason to delay surgery. Ms. C scheduled the procedure for the next week. Because no preoperative general medical tests were required, she reported to the hospital only a short time before the surgery. The only anesthetic is numbing drops like those used during the complete medical eye examination. She had already taken the mild tranquilizer that the ophthalmologist prescribed to ease her nervousness.

The laser surgery was performed at the biomicroscope, with Ms. C sitting on a stool and resting her chin in the chin rest. She had to cooperate during the procedure by looking at various fixation targets as instructed. This moved her eye to give the surgeon access to various areas as required but ensured that it remained stationary at all other times.

The laser cuts a small section out of the periphery of the iris, permitting aqueous fluid to flow out of the anterior chamber at that site. The entire procedure took only 15 to 30 minutes, and when it was over, Ms. C sat in the waiting room and was called back to the examining room periodically to have the pressure in the operated eye checked. Sometimes pressure can elevate right after the procedure, requiring administration of pressure-lowering medication. Once the doctor was satisfied that things were under control and the pressure was in a reasonable range, her eye was patched and she was allowed to go home.

Patching is not essential, but it will make the eye slightly more comfortable since it prevents blinking, a possible irritant to the slightly inflamed eye. Patching will also shield the eye from light, to which it is somewhat sensitive for a few hours after the procedure.

As instructed, Ms. C saw the doctor at the office the next day. The patch was removed and her pressure checked.

The laser treatment had been a success. Although the patient still needed mild eyedrops in the operated eye, pressure could be maintained without the same strength required before the surgery; the right eye, of course, continued to be treated as before.

Four years later the left eye again showed increased tension, inadequately controlled by even the highest-strength medication. The visual field in that eye also showed further loss and there was some increase in the cupping of its optic disc. A second laser procedure was done on the left eye.

Seven years since the original diagnosis, Ms. C has had two laser treatments on the left eye and lost some additional visual field in it, but she still has good visual acuity since her central vision was unaffected. Whereas some people may experience similarly elevated pressure or difficulty with control in both eyes, Ms. C was not unusual in having her right eye remain well controlled, with no additional visual field loss.

Surgical Options

Like medical therapy, glaucoma surgery is directed at either improving the aqueous outflow or decreasing the aqueous secretion. The procedures that mechanically increase the outflow are referred to as *filtration procedures,* and they increase the area from which the fluid flows out of the anterior chamber.

Depending on need, one eye or both can be operated on. As in cataract surgery, however, both eyes are never done at the same time to avoid severe visual impairment should any complications arise.

Trabeculectomy

In effect, a *trabeculectomy* removes a section of the abnormal fibrous tissue in the anterior chamber angle to unclog the drainage mechanism. Even when there is no abnormal tissue, drainage can be improved by cutting into a canal located in the trabecular meshwork. This is called a *trabeculotomy*.

Trabeculoplasty

The procedure done on Ms. C is a *trabeculoplasty*, a procedure using a laser to remove trabecular tissue in an attempt to improve drainage.

Iridectomy

Depending on the anatomical picture presented by the gonioscope, an *iridectomy* can be performed, with laser or iris scissors. Cutting a hole into the periphery of the iris permits aqueous fluid to flow out of the anterior chamber at that site. The tiny hole is covered by the upper eyelid, so it is visible only on close examination and does not let in additional light or in any other way cause discomfort.

Laser Surgery

Laser surgery is one of the great advances in ophthalmology. Before these directed beams of high-intensity light were developed, glaucoma surgery required opening the eye with a surgical instrument and cutting away parts of the internal eye anatomy in an attempt to control the pressure flow. Now a laser beam can often do what a surgical knife did before. Laser types and techniques are constantly undergoing changes in this still-evolving method of therapy.

Laser surgery in general is safer than conventional knife

surgery because it is less invasive: The eye is not opened. It can be done in a doctor's office that is equipped with the appropriate laser or in a hospital on an outpatient basis. Only a local anesthetic is required. It is quick—usually taking about 15 to 30 minutes as compared to a full hour with conventional surgery. Recovery time and the likelihood of complications are decreased, as is postoperative discomfort, because no incision and no stitches are involved.

Patients sometimes experience a transient blurring of vision after a laser procedure because of a slight inflammatory reaction inside the eye. This is normal—after all, the laser acts as a burning knife inside the eye, and the body will definitely react to this insult.

The main complications of laser glaucoma surgery are pronounced inflammation in the eye, bleeding, the development of a secondary cataract or worsening of an existing one, and failure to control or even reduce intraocular pressure.

Knife Surgery

At times laser surgery may not work, or the anatomical situation may require more extensive cutting than lasers permit. In such cases, intraocular knife surgery can be tried. If a cataract is causing the glaucoma, the cataract extraction procedure, which includes as a matter of course a peripheral iridectomy, might be expanded to include a trabeculectomy, the removal of some of the fibrous tissue blocking drainage.

Intraocular glaucoma surgery is done in a hospital, generally under local anesthesia. Most of the time an overnight stay is required.

The main complications are infection, bleeding, failure

to control the glaucoma, and the development of a secondary cataract or the worsening of an existing one.

Trephine

This is a filtration procedure that involves using a very sharp circular punch (a *trephine*) to cut a tiny hole in the sclera at the point where it meets the cornea. This point on the outside of the eye is just above the drainage angle on the inside. The hole becomes a secondary drain for aqueous fluid, which flows under the conjunctiva and is absorbed.

Iridencleisis

Iridencleisis involves cutting a slit in the sclera and trapping a bit of iris tissue in it to make a wicklike opening through which the aqueous fluid can flow and escape under the conjunctiva.

In both of these procedures, the surgical site is small and usually hidden by the upper eyelid. They are not disfiguring or uncomfortable in any way. These procedures were the predominant ones used in the middle of this century, but they have largely been replaced by lasers, which have gained favor very much because they involve less trauma to the eye.

Cryotherapy and Cyclodiathermy

Applying cold *(cryotherapy)* or heat *(cyclodiathermy)* to the ciliary body to reduce secretion of aqueous fluid is another surgical approach. Probes are applied externally, and no incision is required in either method. These procedures can be done under local anesthetic in an ophthalmologist's office or on an outpatient basis at a hospital. Fairly severe inflammation is a usual side effect, and the final results are often disappointing. Because these two methods are not nearly as effective as laser and knife surgery, they are performed less often. Still, they may be tried as a minor procedure in the hope of avoiding more major surgery.

Postsurgical Management

Whether it is necessary to continue antiglaucoma eyedrops after surgery will vary from patient to patient. Often some form of medical therapy will still be necessary. As with Ms. C, a laser procedure may work to control pressure for a while, just as a particular medication does, but then lose its effectiveness. To remedy this, it is certainly possible to repeat a laser procedure at a future time.

We cannot speak of glaucoma as being "cured," but only "controlled." Therefore, once an individual is diagnosed with glaucoma, regular ophthalmological checkups and, in all likelihood, daily eyedrops must become a lifelong commitment. Most patients will agree that this is a worthwhile, minor annoyance. Untreated glaucoma usually ends in blindness, but if it is diagnosed and treated early enough, visual impairment can usually be avoided and eye health and good vision maintained throughout life.

Other Common
Diseases of the Eye

◇

MYTH: A sty results from a cold in the eye, so it is a kind of contagious cold sore.

FACT: A sty is not contagious and it is never caused by a virus, as colds are. *Cold sore* is a common name for an infection of the *herpes simplex* virus. It is possible to get a herpes simplex infection in the eye, but the result will not be a sty, which is a bacterial infection of a gland in the eyelid margin.

MYTH: People who care about the health of their eyes should avoid wearing eye makeup.

FACT: Properly applied, eye makeup will not endanger the health of your eyes. If care is taken to avoid bacterial contamination of your eye makeup (it should not be shared with others, and you should always discard mascara and applicators after two to three months), there is no reason to avoid using these products.

MYTH: Rolling or crossing the eyes is a bad idea because it can make a person cross-eyed.

FACT: Although many of the causes of strabismus (cross-eye) are not well understood, there is absolutely no evidence that rolling, crossing, or in any other way using the eyes or external eye muscles ever causes this condition. These muscles are meant to be used. Rolling the eyes is not very attractive and it may tire the eyes, but it is not at all harmful.

MYTH: Dyslexia, a common learning disability, is caused by problems having to do with the way eye muscles work, and special visual training can solve those problems and cure the dyslexia.

FACT: Dyslexia is connected with how the brain processes written material. It is not a primary vision problem, and true dyslexia is not very common.

MYTH: It is a good idea to eat carrots and other sources of vitamin A because they improve the ability to see in the dark.

FACT: Although it is true that photochemical changes take place in the retina to permit vision in the dark, and that the retina uses vitamin A for this purpose, the amount of vitamin A in a normal, reasonably balanced diet supplies more than enough for such needs. In fact, there is some danger in taking extremely large doses of vitamin A.

MYTH: People who are color-blind see only in black and white.

FACT: Although dogs, cats, and many other animals see in black and white, color-blind people do see colors. They perceive colors less vividly than those with normal color vision, but their world is never completely mono-chromatic.

MYTH: Poor vision in the dark is a sure sign of night blindness, which is a common problem.
FACT: Night blindness is not at all common. Rather, it is a symptom of a rare condition called *retinitis pigmentosa.* Most people have more difficulty seeing at night simply because the lower the light level, the harder it is to see. This is not the same thing as night blindness.

Although cataracts and glaucoma are the most common serious eye diseases encountered by people over the age of 40, eyes are subject to other disorders and injuries requiring medical attention and treatment.

The External Eye

If our eyes are our windows on the world, they are also a doorway through which infection and foreign bodies can pass. Fortunately, the eye's protective system—the eyelids and eyelashes; the tears; the conjunctiva, sclera, and cor-nea—does an excellent job of guarding the delicate interior of the eyeball from infection and other intrusions. Infec-tions inside the eye, when they do occur, usually come from infections in the body, and they tend to be serious. But as much protection as the outer layers of the eye provide, they are themselves vulnerable.

Common external eye problems are generally not seri-ous. Some of them require no treatment at all and go away by themselves; many others are easy for an eye doctor to treat with special medication. If you find yourself with any of the symptoms described in the following pages, do not make your own diagnosis and run to the local pharmacy for over-the-counter medication. See an eye doctor who can properly diagnose and treat the condition to ensure that it does not become a serious eye problem.

Conjunctivitis

Conjunctivitis, commonly known as pinkeye, is used to describe any inflammation of the conjunctiva, the transparent membrane that covers the front surface of the eyeball and laps over onto the inner eyelids. The three main types of conjunctivitis, each named for the cause of the inflammation, are infectious, allergic, and chemical.

Infectious conjunctivitis can be caused by bacteria or by a virus. In both cases, the symptoms are red eyes, inflammation of the inner eyelids, excessive tearing, and a sandy or scratchy feeling in the eyes. People with pinkeye also commonly have a discharge from their eyes that makes the eyelids sticky in the morning, because the discharge is not blinked away during sleep. If the cause of the pinkeye is a bacterial infection, the discharge will be more puslike; if a virus is responsible, the discharge will be more watery.

Bacterial conjuctivitis is treated with antibiotic eyedrops, ointment, or both, all of which must be prescribed by a doctor. Viral conjunctivitis, like all viral infections, cannot be cured with antibiotics. The body's own defense system will work against the virus and in time it should go away. A few antiviral drugs have been developed for specific viruses— herpes, for example. If the virus is identified as one for which medication is available, it will be prescribed. Otherwise, ophthalmologists often prescribe antibiotics to pre-

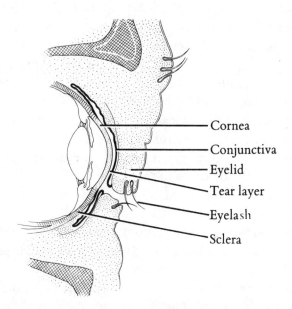

Fig. 9.1   The protective system of the eyeball

vent secondary bacterial infection, since the conjunctiva is more susceptible to bacteria when it is under viral attack.

Infectious pinkeye is contagious, so a few commonsense measures are needed to prevent its spread: People with pinkeye should wash their hands before and after applying eye medication, never share their eyedrops with someone else, keep their hands away from their eyes, and be careful not to share towels or washcloths with others in their household.

Pinkeye can also result from an allergic reaction, and in this case it is not contagious. Anything that can cause an allergic reaction elsewhere in the body—such as pollen, cosmetics, cats, dogs, or fabrics—can cause *allergic conjunctivitis*. The symptoms are itching and burning eyes, pronounced redness, and excessive tearing.

The ideal treatment is to remove the cause of the allergy. If this is impossible—either because it cannot be identified or because you cannot bear to get rid of your cat, for instance—an eye doctor can prescribe one of a variety of eyedrops to help alleviate the symptoms.

Some eyedrops contain a mild local anesthetic, a drug to constrict the blood vessels in the eye and thus to reduce redness, and a soothing liquid. Other kinds of drops contain cortisone, which reduces inflammation. Still others contain cromolyn sodium, which inhibits the allergic reaction. There are also a number of over-the-counter eyedrops that are advertised as effective against allergies, but these are of little use. The medication they offer is quite mild, and they often contain other substances that, although not damaging to the eyes, are not at all effective against allergic conjunctivitis.

Unfortunately, medical science has not been very successful in finding a cure for allergies, so the most widely accepted approach is to try to relieve the discomfort they cause. This is particularly important when the allergy affects the conjunctiva, because rubbing the itchy, irritated eyes will only aggravate the condition. If you are bothered by allergic eye irritation, see your doctor, not your druggist.

Chemical or *toxic conjunctivitis* is caused by irritants in the external environment. These can range from an irritant in a contact lens solution to high levels of air pollution, noxious fumes, or chlorine in swimming pools. As with allergies, the ideal treatment is removal of the irritant. If this is not feasible, lubricating eyedrops to soothe the eyes can be tried. If, for example, you work in a factory where you are constantly exposed to irritating fumes, or if you live in an area with a great deal of smog, nonprescription eyedrops— the kind referred to as *artificial tears*—may be helpful. If highly chlorinated water irritates your eyes, try wearing goggles when you swim.

Sties

The common sty is simply an infection of one of the small glands that lie along the eyelid margin. It is similar to the skin infection known as acne. Sties first appear as painful red lumps on the edge of the eyelid, and in their later stages a head of whitish pus will appear. If sties occur often, some unnoticed chronic infection of the eyelid may be the cause.

Sties are treated with hot compresses applied to the affected area. A clean washcloth dampened with hot tap water is as effective an anything else, although you may use a boric acid solution if you like. In addition, many doctors prescribe antibiotic eyedrops or ointment to control the infection. If this treatment is begun early, it will in most cases clear up the sty in a couple of days. Only rarely will surgical incision and drainage of a sty be required, and when it is, this can be done in an eye doctor's office. Under no circumstances should a sty be squeezed or self-treated with acne medication.

Sties occur more frequently among schoolchildren than among adults. This is not, as might be assumed, because children tend to pick up infections in school. Sties are not contagious and cannot be passed from person to person. Rather, it is more likely because a child's glandular secretions are more erratic, particularly during puberty, and because children tend to be less careful than adults about keeping their hands clean and away from their eyes.

Corneal Infections

The cornea, that clear tissue layer that lies in front of the iris, can become infected in several ways. If its surface is broken by some direct injury—a foreign object that has become lodged in the cornea; a scratch from a paper edge, tree branch, or the sharp edge of a leaf; or an abrasion caused by a fingernail, cosmetic brush, or improper use of contact lenses—a secondary infection can result. Some common corneal infections begin as a complication of pinkeye. Since the cornea is surrounded by the conjunctiva, an untreated infection of the conjunctiva can easily spread to the cornea.

Herpes and chlamydia, two sexually transmitted organisms that have recently come to increased public attention, can infect the cornea as well as other parts of the body. This may occur in babies who are born to women with one of these diseases. Because they are potentially serious corneal infections, they require medical treatment at once.

Older people may suffer more corneal infections than they did when they were younger. Normally our tears provide protection against corneal infection. In the course of the day, the eyes are constantly bathed with tear fluid and our eyelids act as windshield wipers every time we blink. But some people—and all of us to a degree when we get older—secrete less tear fluid. When this happens, the cornea becomes somewhat more susceptible to infection from bacteria or viruses.

The symptoms of corneal infection are pain, which is sometimes severe; a teary, reddened eye that is sensitive to light; a scratchy feeling when you blink. Corneal infections are usually not contagious.

Antibiotic eyedrops and/or ointment are used to treat bacterial infections, and may be prescribed to prevent secondary bacterial infections when a virus is primarily responsible. If the virus is one of those for which specific antiviral drops are available, they will be prescribed.

Often the infected eye is patched to keep it closed; this avoids further irritation and discomfort caused by the eyelid moving over the cornea with every blink.

A corneal infection can also be a secondary result of a corneal burn, often caused by an ultraviolet sunlamp or tanning bed. This is yet another reason to avoid these hazardous devices. The burn itself is extremely painful and needs to be treated medically: with anesthetic drops to relieve the pain and antibiotic drops to guard against secondary infection. And, again, the affected eye is usually patched to give it a rest. If the corneas in both eyes are burned, the doctor may try to patch only one eye so the temporary visual impairment is not total, but in some cases both eyes must be patched.

Scleritis

The white of the eye can become inflamed, usually in response to infections or irritations in adjacent tissues. Less frequently, the inflammation originates with the sclera itself. When it does, this is called *scleritis,* and it is most often the result of an allergic reaction and, therefore, is not contagious. A much rarer scleritis can be caused by infection in the white of the eye. The symptoms of true scleritis are a reddened sclera and slight discomfort; it is usually treated with eyedrops containing cortisone.

Blepharitis

Blepharitis is an infection of the glands of the eyelid margins. It bears a similarity to dandruff, and it often occurs in people who have dandruff of the scalp as well. It is usually a chronic condition, which means it tends to recur, yet it is often present in a very mild form, with minor, if any, symptoms. It can also appear in an acute form, at which time the infection is active and the symptoms are quite obvious. People with acute blepharitis have reddened and encrusted eyelid margins. The treatment for this is an eyedrop containing cortisone and an antibiotic. Many doctors also prescribe an effective antidandruff shampoo for the scalp and eyebrows, and instruct patients to clean their lashes and eyelid margins with either a "no-tears" baby shampoo or a special cleaning formula designed for the purpose. People who have chronic blepharitis and suffer recurrent attacks should use the shampoo and clean their eyelid margins preventively, three times a week or more, even when the condition is inactive.

Blepharitis is not contagious, and it is usually mild and easy to treat. If it is severe or neglected, however, abscesses of the eyelids, secondary infections of other parts of the eye, and loss of the eyelashes may result.

Chalazions

A *chalazion* is a cyst inside the eyelid caused by an infection. The infected cyst is painful and reddish; when the infection goes away, the cyst remains as a painless lump. The treatment for an infected chalazion is the application of hot compresses (using a clean washcloth and hot tap water) and antibiotic drops or ointment. This will make the infection subside, but the cyst itself will go away only in rare cases.

Once the acute infection has cleared up, the chalazion may have to be removed surgically. This is a minor operation that can be done with local anesthetic in the eye doctor's office, and it leaves no noticeable scar. Although this is never an emergency operation and there is no danger that the cyst will become malignant, most opthalmologists will remove chalazions because they tend to become reinfected.

Recurrent chalazions can be caused by an undetected chronic eyelid infection or by muscle pressure on the eyelid glands. Chalazions are not contagious.

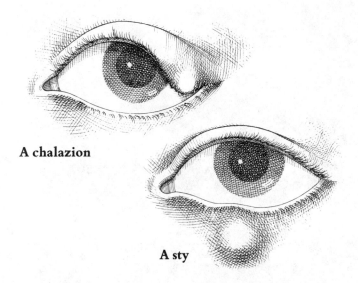

A chalazion

A sty

Fig. 9.2

Subconjunctival Hemorrhage

A common and frightening eye problem that is not at all serious is a burst blood vessel in the eye. It is called a *subconjunctival hemorrhage* and is really just like a bruise anywhere else on the body. One of the tiny blood vessels in the eye bursts and blood seeps between the conjunctiva and the sclera. Because the conjunctiva is clear, the blood looks bright red instead of black and blue, as it commonly appears when beneath a layer of skin. A subconjunctival hemorrhage may cause a large red area in the eye, but because it is completely painless, it is most often noticed by someone else.

The hemorrhage may be caused by trauma to the eye, but it usually happens completely spontaneously, and there is

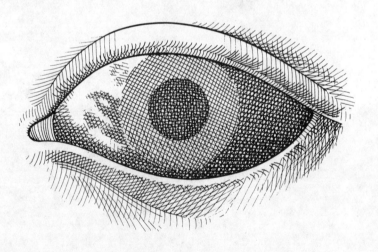

Fig. 9.3   A subconjunctival hemorrhage

no treatment for it. The blood will be gradually reabsorbed in the course of 10 to 14 days. There is nothing effective that you can do to make it go away faster, but it is nothing to worry about. This condition does not suggest any underlying illness of the eye or any sort of circulatory problem.

Eyelid Tics

Another problem that patients often complain about is a twitching of the eyelid. This is not a medical eye problem, although it can be a nuisance, because people feel self-conscious about the twitch and are certain others can notice it. Although it feels very obvious, the twitch is barely perceptible. It is caused by *fibrillation,* or quivering, of the muscles around the eye, invariably the result of tension or anxiety. It is not any kind of eye disease or eye muscle disorder.

The problem often vanishes once the patient understands that the cause is tension rather than a potentially serious physical problem. Ignoring the tic, and feeling confident that it is not grossly visible to others, is the most effective therapy.

Ptosis

Abnormal drooping of the upper eyelid can occur for a variety of reasons. It may be present at birth, either as a result of a problem during fetal formation or an actual birth injury. It can be of neurological origin, indicating a defect or injury to the nerve that supplies the upper eyelid, or it can result from trauma to the eyelid itself. If the condition is so severe that the pupil is covered and vision impaired, plastic surgery can be done to lift the eyelid.

Cosmetic Eye Surgery

As we age, all of our body tissues tend to lose their resiliency: Our skin wrinkles and our muscles become less firm. These changes are especially noticeable around the eyes, and because the eyes play such a major role in an individual's appearance (or at least one's own feelings about it), cosmetic eye surgery is increasingly pondered once those lines, wrinkles, and puffiness around the eyes become more pronounced.

Although such cosmetic surgery is not necessarily dangerous, important considerations should govern the decision to embark on this elective procedure.

Whenever knife, scissors, and sutures are used, there is a danger of complications: infection, excessive bleeding, and the formation of abnormal, disfiguring scars. Plastic surgery, by its nature, alters the natural anatomical relationships of skin with its underlying tissues and muscles. Keep in mind that cosmetic eye surgery is an attempt either to remove bags from the upper and/or lower eyelids or to decrease wrinkles; it tightens the skin and muscles around the eye, and to obtain this tightening effect, skin and muscle must be removed.

Dry Eyes

As a result of cosmetic eye surgery, the functioning of the blink reflex is virtually always affected. Diminution of this reflex and the consequent decrease in adequate distribution of tears over the cornea often result in irritable eyes, especially if dry eyes due to decreased tear production was already a problem. This is of particular relevance to contact lens wearers, who may experience discomfort and, in some cases, find they are unable to wear their lenses at all after surgery. Even for those who do not wear lenses, the symptoms of reduced tear production that almost everyone experiences with age are exacerbated after cosmetic eye surgery. This often leads to redder and more irritable eyes that may also be more prone to infection.

Repeat Procedures

Although most plastic repairs result in improvement, many must be repeated in five to ten years. This is necessary because further aging and slackening of the skin will now result in an appearance that is worse than what would have occurred with no surgery at all.

For any surgical procedure, doctor and patient must consider the risk/benefit ratio. For cosmetic surgery, in which definite risk is balanced against a subjective benefit, a long, hard, and candid look is warranted. In some instances, a psychiatric consultation may be of use to help clarify motives and expectations in the face of the risks. In any case, no one should have cosmetic eye surgery without insisting that the surgeon clearly outline all the potential risks and complications in addition to the expected cosmetic outcome.

Retinal Disorders

The retina is the delicate, thin structure often compared to the film of a camera. It is responsible for receiving visual messages—what we see—and sending them to the brain by way of the optic nerve. The ability to see colors is part of the function of the retina, as is the ability to see well in different levels of light. In order to do its work, the retina should not be scarred or torn, and nothing should interfere with the work of its tiny blood vessels. No blood should be present anywhere in the retina except in those blood vessels. Furthermore, the adhesion of the retina to the two structures that lie on either side of it—the choroid and the vitreous fluid—must not be interrupted.

When any one of these conditions is not fulfilled, vision can be affected. The seriousness of the effect depends on where on the retina the problem exists. If it is out on the far edges—that part of the retina that receives peripheral visual information—it is unlikely that there will be any noticeable loss of vision. However, the closer to the center the problem lies, the more noticeable it will be. Moreover, any damage to the macular area—the specialized area of the retina that provides sharp, central vision—will be very noticeable indeed.

Diagnosing Retinal Disorders

The prime instrument for diagnosing retinal disorders is the ophthalmoscope, which permits an ophthalmologist to view the retina directly. Because everything that lies in front of the retina—the cornea, aqueous fluid, lens, and vitreous fluid—are transparent, direct examination of this internal structure is possible. It is even possible to examine part of the circulatory system, and this is often a valuable tool in diagnosing diseases elsewhere in the body that affect vascular health.

Other diagnostic procedures include *fluorescein angiography* and fundus photography. Fluorescein angiography is done by injecting a dye into a blood vessel of the arm, which carries it to the retina. The dye will show up in photographs of the retina, outlining its circulation and showing any abnormalities that may exist. This can be very useful, for example, when diabetes is damaging retinal circulation. Fundus photographs of the retina are taken with equipment similar to that used to photograph the optic disc in glaucoma. The purpose is the same, too: to obtain a permanent visual record that documents the progression of any retinal problem.

Visual field testing is another diagnostic tool with applications for eye disorders other than glaucoma. Any interference along the pathways between the optic nerve and the visual center of the brain can cause problems that will be reflected in the visual field. Among the possible interferences are infections, allergic reactions, and increased pressure on the brain caused by mechanical or circulatory factors.

It is particularly fortunate that one or more characteristics of the visual field abnormality will often tell the ophthalmologist the location of a lesion along the pathways from the optic nerve to the brain, the density and size of the lesion, and through medical experience, even what the probable cause is. Just as we have seen that there are characteristic visual field defects in glaucoma, there are also such characteristic visual field defects for certain types of brain tumors, for strokes, for brain inflammation or infections, for neurological diseases like multiple sclerosis or amyotrophic lateral sclerosis, and for many other conditions that obstruct the visual pathway. Finally, localized problems in the eye itself, such as retinal detachment, macular degeneration, retinal pigmentary disturbances, tumors inside the eyeball, or scar tissue in the retina from infection or circulatory problems, will cause visual field defects, many of which can be quite characteristic of the underlying medical problem.

Retinal Detachment

One of the most serious retinal problems occurs when something interferes with the adherence of the retina to the choroid, and the retina pulls away. The possible causes for this are numerous, some well known and others not. Torn retinal tissue can cause detachment, or detachment itself can cause the retina to tear. Other causes can be a blow to the eye, a cyst or tumor, scar tissue, a hemorrhage, infection, or some other disease of the eye. It could even simply be a general tendency toward poor adhesion. In rare cases severe nearsightedness can predispose to detachment. And as we know, retinal detachment can be a complication of cataract surgery.

A detached retina does not hurt. Symptoms include visual loss (especially in one area of the visual field), spots before the eyes, and light flashes. But this does not mean that anyone who experiences these symptoms has a detached retina. If you notice such problems with your eyes, see your eye doctor as soon as possible to identify the cause and begin appropriate treatment, if necessary.

Retinal detachment is serious. For one thing, it will nearly always get worse if it is not treated quickly. The detached area tends to get larger, or the retina may tear away in several places. Wherever the detachment occurs, the retinal tissue no longer functions as it should and some sight is lost.

The treatment of retinal detachment is always surgical. The aim is to reattach the retina and do everything possible to make sure it does not detach again. When the underly-

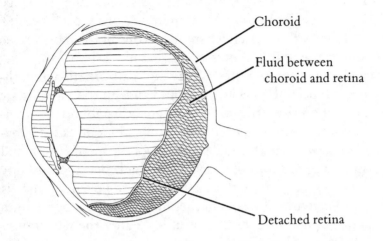

Choroid

Fluid between
choroid and retina

Detached retina

Fig. 9.4   Retinal detachment

ing cause is known, it too can be treated. But often the cause
is not known or, as in severe nearsightedness, it is incurable.
   There are a number of ways to repair a retinal detachment, none of which leaves a visible scar or requires cutting
into the eye itself. Cryotherapy and cyclodiathermy, the
cold and heat probes applied to the ciliary body in an
attempt to decrease aqueous secretion in glaucoma, also
have an application here. Applied to the sclera, these cause
scar formation around a retinal tear or hole, which therefore seals the area. Sometimes lasers are used to cauterize
the tear. Again, no incision is involved; the laser beam is
aimed through the pupil. Another procedure shortens the
eyeball slightly by giving it a tuck in the back portion and
securing it with silicone. Some of the external eye muscles

may be cut to give access to the part of the eye being repaired, but they are reattached as soon as the repair has been done. Remember the importance of a second opinion and the fact that laser eye surgery is one of the most abused and overused procedures in ophthalmic surgery.

Surgery on the vitreous may be a part of retinal detachment repair. If abnormal fibrous bands in the vitreous are pulling on the retina, or if there are other abnormal opacities in the vitreous, a microsurgical technique called *vitrectomy* may be performed. This involves fragmenting and aspirating portions of the vitreous fluid. Because the body cannot regenerate vitreous fluid, the removed vitreous is replaced with saline or another fluid substitute. Sometimes actual donor vitreous fluid is utilized after the vitrectomy. This is called a *vitreous implant.*

Unfortunately, the success rate of retinal surgery is not as high as it is with other eye procedures. When it is a success, the retina stays reattached and vision will be unimpaired. Sometimes the retina stays reattached but damage has already been done to the retinal tissue and some vision is thus lost in the damaged area. The degree of the visual impairment depends upon where the detachment took place. If it was on the periphery, little if any visual handicap will result; if it was closer to the center, a greater loss of vision can be expected. In some cases the retina may become detached again. What is frustrating about this is that if the underlying cause cannot be identified or treated, the possibility of a recurrence is increased.

On a positive note, retinal detachment is not at all common. If it is a relatively well-known eye problem, that is probably because of occasional mention in the media of athletes who suffer retinal detachment as a consequence of a sports-related injury. For most people, it simply is not a frequent occurrence.

Vitreous Floaters

The vast majority of people who experience symptoms of spots before their eyes are suffering not from retinal detachment but from *vitreous floaters.* These small conglomerations of cells have been released from the lining of the inside of the eyeball and literally float in the vitreous fluid. They are usually apparent when you look at a white background in certain light levels, and they appear as tiny spots, specks, or doughnut-shaped forms. Vitreous floaters are not a disease, though they can be a nuisance. They tend to occur more in nearsighted people and, although they can be recurrent, they most often are reabsorbed and disappear on their own. There is no effective treatment for vitreous floaters, and the best thing to do is to try to ignore the minor annoyance they can cause.

There are a number of other conditions that affect the retina. Some can cause detachment or other, less serious problems. Some can be treated, some go away by themselves, and some can be left alone.

Retinal Hemorrhage

A hemorrhage is simply the term for a break in a blood vessel. This can occur in various parts of the body and can be caused for a number of different reasons. When it takes place in the retina, the blood interferes with the function of the retinal cells that are receiving visual stimuli. In most cases a hemorrhage will actually take care of itself: The break in the vessel will seal and the blood will be reabsorbed and carried away as waste. In that case, partial loss of vision, if indeed there is any, is usually temporary. In other cases, the hemorrhage may leave fibrous scar tissue that will inter- fere with the work of the retinal cells. That part of the ret- ina will not be able to receive or send visual information. Depending on where the scar is, the loss of vision may be serious, minor, or unnoticeable. However, the most serious danger of a retinal hemorrhage is when scar tissue pulls at the retina and causes it to detach. Although retinal hem- orrhages can have serious consequences, they are often quite minor. A retinal hemorrhage that does not interfere with vision may go unnoticed until an ophthalmologist observes distintive scarring on the retina.

If the reason for a retinal hemorrhage cannot be explained, the patient should be examined for general cir- culatory problems in order to rule those out.

Retinal Infections

Like all other tissues in the body, the retina is susceptible to infection. The source of infection is usually somewhere else in the body, and the blood carries the infectious agents to the retina. Such varied conditions as tuberculosis, parasites, syphilis, and viruses such as herpes and cytomegalovirus (a common infection in AIDS patients) can infect the retina. The best treatment is to cure the underlying infection whenever possible. If your eye doctor notices certain infec- tions while examining your eyes, he or she may refer you to your family doctor. Your eye doctor and family doctor can then work together to try to discover the underlying infection. In the best circumstances, the infection can be cleared up with no loss of vision. In some cases, retinal tissue in certain areas will be damaged and will no longer function. And, in very serious cases, the scarring caused by the infection could bring on a retinal detachment.

Other Retinal Disorders

A blow to the eye can cause injury to the retina, provoking a hemorrhage, swelling, or even detachment. In most cases, the injury is minor and temporary, but it can be serious. If you are struck in the eye and notice blurring or spots before your eyes, or a partial loss of vision, see an ophthalmologist right away.

Much rarer retinal problems are tumors and cysts, but these are usually benign. Depending on their size and location on the retina, growths can cause partial loss of vision and detachment. Treatment will be determined by the cause, location, and character of the tumor or cyst.

Color Blindness

Color blindness is an untreatable condition of the retina that is not very well understood. Doctors suspect an abnormality in the specialized cells of the retina that are responsible for the perception of color, but the exact problem is unknown. We do know that color blindness is hereditary and occurs almost exclusively in men, although it can be genetically transmitted through women. Also, color blindness is present at birth and never develops later in life, nor can it get better or worse with age.

Color blindness can be slight or severe. In general, though, the color-blind person can adjust to the problem and "perceive" colors from other visual clues. In no case does a color-blind person see only in black and white. Usually, he will simply have a less vivid perception of a certain color or colors and be able to perceive a narrower range of shadings. Obviously, color blindness is a serious handicap for someone who works in the visual arts or other fields requiring exact and specific perception of colors, but for most color-blind people, it is a minor handicap to which one can easily adjust.

The Retina and Circulatory Diseases

One of the nicest things about the retina is that it is very easy to examine. And because the retina is the only place in the whole body where living blood vessels are visible for direct examination, it may provide clues in the diagnosis of a particular group of circulatory ailments also affecting the retinal blood circulation. In all cases the treatment is aimed toward the condition as a whole rather than the retina alone.

Arteriosclerosis

Arteriosclerosis is often referred to as "hardening of the arteries," but the term is misleading since the arteries do not become hard but merely clogged with fatty deposits; they are less elastic, providing narrower passageways for the blood. The overall effect of arteriosclerosis is therefore less-efficient circulation of the blood.

Under normal conditions, arteriosclerosis is a result of advancing age. As we grow older, we will all develop "hardening of the arteries" to some degree. But arterio-sclerosis can also occur prematurely. There are various causes for this, among them diabetes and, many experts believe, high-fat diets or at least the inability to metabolize fats properly.

This affects the eye and the retina in particular because if the arteries throughout the body are becoming clogged, the arteries of the retina are no exception. Retinal circulation slows down, the delicate cells of the retina are not so effectively fed and washed by the blood, and the cells begin to die. When a retinal cell dies, one fewer cell is available to receive and transmit visual information. How much this affects vision depends again on the location of the dead cell. If it lies on the far periphery of the retina, it corresponds to peripheral vision, and any loss of sight will probably not be noticed. If, however, such a cell is near the macula, sharp

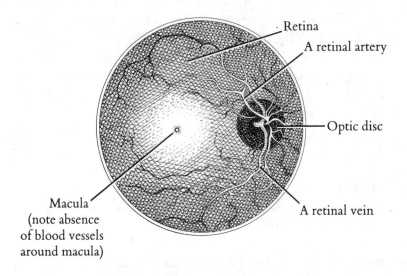

Fig. 9.5   Retinal circulation

central vision can be decreased, and that will be very notice-able indeed. Arteriosclerosis is a progressive disease that causes increased clogging and greater death of retinal cells. In severe cases visual loss may result.

The management of arteriosclerosis should be under-taken by the family doctor. There is no effective way for an eye doctor to treat the circulatory problem as it relates to the retina exclusively, but if an individual is for some reason unaware of having arteriosclerosis, an eye doctor will be able to diagnose it during a regular checkup by looking at the circulation of the retina. He or she will then refer the patient to the family doctor.

Hypertension

Hypertension, or high blood pressure, is another condition that affects the entire body and can show up in the retinal circulation. The effect on the retina occurs only if the hypertension is severe and has not been treated until an advanced stage. When that has happened, hemorrhages may occur and interfere with vision. Fibrous scar tissue left by a hemorrhage can pull at the retina and cause more hem-orrhages, which lead to additional scarring and eventual detachment.

Diabetes

A relatively common condition, diabetes is a metabolic dis-order in which the body does not produce enough insulin to process the sugar it needs. Although it is incurable, dia-betes can be controlled quite successfully with various drugs, injections of insulin, and changes in diet. Very seri-ous, uncontrolled, or undetected cases of diabetes, how-ever, do damage to the blood vessels of the entire body. One result is premature arteriosclerosis. A more serious effect is a condition called *diabetic retinopathy,* a cycle of retinal hemorrhaging followed by scarring, then the abnormal proliferation of tiny blood vessels in the scar tissue, and more hemorrhaging. Diabetic retinopathy is one of the leading causes of blindness today. Although an eye doctor will be able to say that the eye problem is the result of advanced or badly controlled diabetes, treatment must be aimed at the whole condition, not just the effects on the retina. This is just another reason for careful control of diabetes.

Macular Degeneration

This is a condition that can cause some permanent loss of eyesight, although it virtually never leads to complete blindness. It is a common cause of visual loss in patients over sixty. Macular degeneration usually starts in one eye and only later may affect the other. Its main symptom is visual distortion.

There are three forms of macular degeneration: a dry form (90 percent of cases), a wet form (5–10 percent of cases), and the rarest form—*pigment epithelial detachment* (under 5 percent of cases). The dry form is most commonly caused by aging and its associated arteriosclerosis. Examination of the retina by ophthalmoscopy, as well as special studies such as fluorscein angiography and fundus photography, will determine the type. There is no effective medical or surgical treatment for the dry or the pigment epithelial types. In the wet type, abnormal blood vessels grow under the retina and can cause retinal bleeding. In this type laser surgery may be beneficial, not in improving symptoms but in arresting them. The laser causes scar tissue, tending to seal the blood vessels and preventing them from causing further bleeding. However, new blood vessels often grow again after laser treatment, and at times laser surgery can even worsen the condition.

Most of us will never experience any eye problems related to the retina. But all of us should bear in mind that these problems can be serious when they arise. It is fortunate that the retina lends itself so well to examination. All that remains is for you to make yourself regularly available for a periodic eye exam.

Commonsense Eye Care:
How to Spend the Least
to Get the Best

◇

MYTH: Reading or watching television in bad light can ruin your eyes.
FACT: The quality and level of light used for reading, watching television, or in any way using your eyes has no effect on your eyesight or eye health. Although it is easier and more comfortable to read in an adequately illuminated area, it is comfort, not eye health, that should decide how we read a magazine or watch TV.

MYTH: It is a good idea to wash your eyes regularly with eyewash.
FACT: The tears naturally produced by the eyes are the best and only eyewash necessary. They lubricate the eyes and wash away pollutants with every blink.

MYTH: Fluorescent lighting is bad for the eyes because of the ultraviolet radiation it emits.

FACT: There are no health dangers or benefits to be derived from either fluorescent or incandescent light. Fluorescent lighting does not represent a source of dangerous ultraviolet radiation, although natural sunlight in fact does. People who work in areas lit by fluorescent light will be wasting their money if they spend it on UV-coated glasses for indoor wear.

MYTH: Children should have their first eye examination when they enter the first grade.

FACT: Every child should have his or her eyes examined by a medical eye doctor at age three. If there are no problems at that time, the next exam can take place at age six. However, if the doctor spots a problem that might interfere with the child's learning to see, it could then be corrected while the child is still young enough to develop normal vision.

MYTH: If you need to see an eye doctor, it does not matter if you see an ophthalmologist, an oculist, an optometrist, or an optician, since they are all more or less the same.

FACT: They are *not* all the same, and it matters greatly which you consult about medical eye care. Opticians are not eye doctors at all; they are technicians who make corrective lenses according to a doctor's prescription. Optometrists are doctors of optometry, not M.D.'s. They are neither trained nor licensed to treat medical eye problems, though they can prescribe corrective lenses. Ophthalmologists are medical eye doctors, trained and licensed to prescribe corrective lenses, treat diseases of the eye, perform eye surgery, and give complete medical eye care. (Oculist is just another name for ophthalmologist.)

MYTH: Getting a second opinion is just another way doctors have of making money. The time and money spent on getting a second opinion is rarely worth it because doctors usually agree anyway.

FACT: A second opinion can be of great value to consumers. It can save you a lot of money and, more important, unnecessary surgery. Insurance carriers often require second opinions before they will pay for elective surgery, even though it involves an extra examination they will have to pay for. It is important to get a second opinion from an ophthalmologist who is not personally or otherwise connected with the one who originally recommended surgery.

Commonsense eye care can be practiced by consumers who understand how the eyes work and what sorts of things can go wrong, through accidents, disease, and aging. It includes getting regular medical eye examinations and working with an ophthalmologist with whom you have a trusting relationship. But there is much consumers can and must do on their own, and that starts with finding an ophthalmologist.

First Aid for Eye Injuries

There are times when eye discomfort or injury is minor and can be treated at home. But to make sure you are not being penny-wise and pound-foolish, you should know what constitutes an emergency requiring immediate medical attention.

True Eye Emergencies

Because the human eye is pretty tough and well protected, there are only four true eye emergencies, cases when sight is endangered and immediate medical care is required.

Acute Glaucoma

The symptoms of an acute glaucoma attack are severe eye pain, pronounced redness of the eye, blurred vision, and possibly abdominal pain and nausea. Do not try to diagnose acute glaucoma yourself. If you experience such symptoms, go immediately to an eye doctor or to a hospital emergency room. Acute glaucoma is quite rare, but it must be attended to without delay to guard against the danger of severe visual loss.

Penetrating Eye Injury

When a high-velocity foreign body enters the eye and pierces its protective layers, sight can be threatened. This does not refer to particles of grit or other airborne bodies that might land on the conjunctiva or cornea, nor does it mean a finger that has been poked into the eye. Although these can be painful, they are not likely to damage your sight. High-speed power equipment in a factory or a workshop may throw off a sharp, hard object traveling at a speed fast enough to pierce the protective layers and enter the interior of the eyeball.

This kind of injury may take place without causing much pain. If the object is tiny and traveling fast enough, the place where it enters the eye may seal up immediately, so that little or no pain will be felt. Nonetheless, it can have catastrophic results and is to be avoided at all costs. Anyone who works with power tools or other high-speed equipment must wear protective goggles. People who have good vision in only one eye are well advised to avoid such situations altogether. If such an injury occurs, you must get to an eye doctor or a hospital emergency room as soon as possible. First-aid measures will only waste time and are of no value in this case.

Severe Bleeding in or Around the Eye

When flying glass or jagged metal has cut the face, severe bleeding may result. (An automobile accident is a common example of this.) While taking steps to get emergency medical treatment, you should also apply first-aid measures. Try to stop the flow of blood by applying pressure to the wounded area with a clean cloth. Do not try this if applying pressure will drive any glass or metal farther into the eye or skin.

Chemical Eye Injury

When a very strong chemical, such as lye, gets into an eye, it is absolutely essential for the eye to be flushed with large quantities of water as soon as possible. Do not wait for a doctor to do this; follow the first-aid instructions for flushing the eye. The time saved can truly be sight-saving.

At-Home Care for Nonemergencies

Aside from the four emergency situations mentioned above, injury to the eye can be treated at home or given first aid before medical attention is sought.

Foreign Particles in the Eye

Perhaps the most common nonemergency eye problem is getting something in the eye. Depending on what and where it is, a speck can be either a minor irritant or very painful. The first thing to do is to remain calm and proceed as quickly as possible to a well-lighted mirror. In the meantime, the eye will be trying to solve the problem on its own by shutting involuntarily and secreting more than the normal amount of tears. Both of these reflexes are beneficial: Shutting the lids avoids scratching the surface of the eyeball, and tears will tend to wash the particle away. In many cases, whatever was in the eye is gone by the time you arrive in front of a mirror.

If the particle is still there, do not rub the eye or try to remove the particle with your fingers. If you can see the

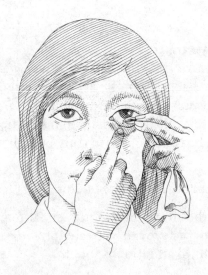

Fig. 10.1   You can try to remove a foreign body from your eye with a clean handkerchief. Do not try it if it is on your cornea.

particle in the mirror, you can try to remove it with the corner of a clean handkerchief or some other clean, lint-free cloth. It may be easier to have someone do this for you, but it is certainly possible to do the job yourself. If you do not have a handkerchief, do not try to remove the particle with a facial tissue or cotton-tipped swab; these will probably introduce other, smaller foreign bodies. And never try to remove a particle in this way unless it is on the white of the eye or on the inner eyelid. The danger of abrasion is simply too great when a particle is on the cornea.

If you cannot see the particle, if it is on the cornea, if you do not have a clean handkerchief, or if you are simply uneasy about poking around in your eye, try to float it off. Fill a sink, bowl, or eye cup with lukewarm tap water and try to open your eye underwater. (If you do not have access to any of these, cup your hand and fill it with water.) If this procedure does not seem to have worked the first time, try it again, moving your eyeball around underwater as much as possible. Although you can use an eyewash for this, it is not necessary and will not be more effective than tap water. If you still feel the particle in your eye, try pulling the upper eyelid over the lower lid. Hold on by the lashes and then quickly release the lid to dislodge the particle. You can try this two or three times.

The particle, and all this poking around the eye, will tend to irritate the eye. In many cases, the particle is long gone even though it still feels as if something were there. Wait a few minutes to see if the irritated feeling goes away. Close your eyes and relax a bit, then blink a few times, letting the tears flow around your eyeball. Close your eyes again. In most cases, the irritation will subside.

Note: Although you may feel the particle in a particular place in your eye—under the upper eyelid on the right side,

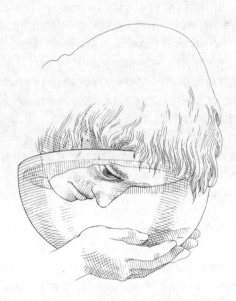

Fig. 10.2   You can try to float a foreign body out of your eye by keeping the eye open underwater.

for example—it may in fact be somewhere else. It is hard to localize a foreign particle accurately. Keep this in mind when you are looking for it and also if a doctor is trying to remove it. Patients will often insist that the doctor is looking in the wrong part of their eye when in fact the doctor *sees* it in a different place from where they think they *feel* it.

If you still feel the particle, and all these attempts have failed to remove it, go to an eye doctor or hospital emergency room.

Chemical in the Eye

A liquid or solid chemical substance in the eye can be a minor irritant or a major catastrophe, as with lye or strong acids. Even if you do not know what the substance is, the first thing to do is to flush the eye quickly and thoroughly with clear water. Do not try to figure out what the substance is and devise an antidote. This will use up precious time. Flushing the eye immediately with lots of water will dilute and wash the substance from the eye, possibly avoiding damage to the eyeball.

The fastest and most effective way to flush the eyes is to rush to the nearest sink, cup your hands, and fill them with water. Hold your hands to your eye and try to open the eye. Meanwhile, permit the sink to fill up so you can put your eyes underwater fast, leaving your hands free to force the

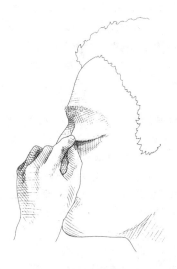

Fig. 10.3 **Sometimes you can dislodge a particle by pulling down and then releasing your upper eyelid.**

lids open. Continue flushing the eyes for several minutes after any pain has subsided. If pain persists, if the eye is red, if there is any loss of vision, or if you know or suspect that the chemical is very strong, grab the container and rush to an eye doctor or hospital emergency room.

Take particular care not to put your hands in or near your eyes when you are working with household chemicals, and be especially careful with aerosols. No matter what the other ingredients are, aerosols always contain propellants that are harmful to the eyes. Hair sprays and spray deodorants commonly find their way into people's eyes. Always close your eyes when you are using these products and keep them closed for a few seconds after you have finished, because the vapors tend to hang in the air. If it is not possible to keep your eyes closed (in the case of spray paints, for example), shield your eyes, keep the can at arm's length, or wear goggles of some sort. And by all means, look to see in what direction the nozzle is pointing before you depress the button!

Burns

If you splash hot oil or hot water into the eyes, the first step is to flush them with cool water. The fact that oil is not soluble in water is irrelevant, since you are trying to flood it out, not dissolve it. Cool water will also tend to reduce the temperature of the burned tissues. If the burn is serious and painful, see a doctor. Do not, under any circumstances, try to apply burn ointments, butter, or anything els intended for skin burns.

An eyelid burn from a sunlamp or from the sun itself no different from a skin burn elsewhere on your bod just may feel more painful since the skin of your lids is tender. In most cases, the irritation will go away in a two, but you can, if you like, apply a commercial sunburn cream or lotion. Be sure to do it carefully, making sure to get nothing in your eyes. Many of these preparations contain mild local anesthetics to relieve discomfort, but they also often contain chemicals that can sting the eyes. A cold compress (a clean washcloth dampened with cold tap water placed over your closed eyelids) or an ice pack may reduce swelling from the burn and cool the skin.

Ultraviolet Radiation

Ultraviolet radiation poses an immediate and long-term danger, whether it comes from the sun or a tanning device. When skin burns, it sustains damage that may eventually result in skin cancer. The eyelids and area around the eyes are very common sites for skin cancer. Apply common sense in protecting this delicate skin: Use sunscreens and sunglasses whenever you are in direct sunlight. Artificial tanning devices—whether commercial tanning booths, beds, or a home sunlamp—can be particularly dangerous because the ultraviolet light they emit is many times more intense than natural sunlight. Most doctors feel they should never be used at all. If you choose to ignore this advice, do not rely on sunglasses and/or sunscreens to protect the eyes. You must use the opaque eye shields that the law requires to be supplied with all artificial tanning devices. Then keep your eyes closed even if your back is to the lamp, because the reflected light is sufficient to cause a burn.

Injury Around the Eyes

Minor cuts near the eyes should be treated like cuts elsewhere on the body. If there is bleeding, apply pressure to the area until the bleeding stops. Use sterile gauze, if available, or a clean handkerchief. If the cut is large or the bleeding continues, seek medical attention. Apply antiseptic and an adhesive bandage strip to small cuts and abrasions, as you would with any cut. Keep the wound clean and protected from additional injury, and take care to keep any antiseptic out of the eye.

A "black eye" is really nothing more than a bruise, showing up bluish-purple at first and then gradually fading in 10 days to two weeks. There is nothing you can do to make it fade faster, and that includes using steak on the area. If you want to try this old folk remedy, be sure to buy a good steak so you can eat it afterward. It will not help your eye, but a juicy steak dinner might cheer you up. Ice will reduce the swelling somewhat.

Fill a sock or washcloth with a few ice cubes, or purchase a commercial ice pack. The type containing a freezable gel—either one use or reusable—may be more comfortable because the pack conforms to the contour of the eye area. Do not keep the ice in contact with the skin for more than a couple of minutes at a time, though you can repeat it as often as you wish with 20-minute intervals in between. You will not do any harm to the eye if you cover the bruise with flesh-colored makeup.

Aspirin can be an effective pain reliever in any of these instances. If you can take aspirin or one of the aspirin substitutes, by all means do so. Two tablets every four hours (for adults), for as long as mild pain relief is needed, should suffice.

Corneal Injuries

Injury to the cornea, regardless of the cause, is more serious than injury to the conjunctiva and other external parts of the eye. This is why you should not attempt to remove a particle from the cornea. If you get something on your cornea and cannot flush or blink it away, have a doctor remove it. And if your cornea becomes scratched or abraded, this too will require medical attention. What you can do in the meantime is to try to keep your eye closed, since the main discomfort is actually caused by blinking. You may wish to devise an eye patch using sterile gauze and adhesive tape. A corneal burn is another painful injury that must be treated by a doctor. There are a number of ways a cornea can become burned, but the most common is from sunlamps, a powerful reason to avoid these and any other artificial tanning devices.

How to Choose an Eye Doctor

Total medical eye care can be provided only by an ophthalmologist, a specialist in eye medicine. As mentioned earlier, optometrists, who are not medical doctors, can prescribe glasses or contact lenses, but they cannot treat eye diseases. In general, the eye care they give is quite limited and, even in the area of prescribing corrective lenses, they are not trained or (in many states) licensed to use any kind of eyedrops, including dilating drops. These particular drops are extremely helpful in determining a prescription with complete accuracy.

If a private ophthalmological examination is beyond your budget, visit an eye clinic at a nearby teaching hospital. Although there will be inconveniences involved, you will be treated by doctors who are being trained in the specialty of ophthalmology and are working under supervision. If there is no such clinic available in your area or if you are reluctant to avail yourself of its services, optometrists are a much less desirable option. Make such a choice, if absolutely necessary, only if you are between the ages of 20 and 40, the period when eye health is least likely to be complicated, require medical attention, or undergo change. This is generally past the time when childhood eye problems and optical changes occur, but before the age when medical eye exams are of greatest value.

One of the reasons people go to optometrists rather than ophthalmologists is that they are attracted by the offer of free or low-cost eye examinations. What they should understand is that optometrists are in the business of selling glasses. In view of the cost of glasses today, a free exam from an optometrist can be very expensive indeed. Although there are certainly many ethical optometrists, many customers are sold glasses that are unnecessary, or they are told they need a change of prescription when they do not. A common example of this is the under-40 nearsighted person who is sold two separate pairs of glasses, one for reading and the other for distance vision. Anyone who understands optical errors will immediately recognize this as a ruse to sell an extra pair of glasses, because virtually no person under 40, who therefore still has near-focusing ability, needs different glasses for near and distance vision. Once the optical error of myopia is corrected with a single pair of glasses, the image comes to focus on the retina (see Figure, page 48). This occurs regardless of the distance of the object being viewed.

Another example of unnecessary expense is the person who is told a slight change in prescription is needed—and while ordering new corrective lenses, why not get new frames? In fact, a minimal change in optics usually does *not* require a new pair of glasses. Some optometrists also prescribe very weak reading glasses for customers under 40 who complain of mild eyestrain and headaches when reading. Consumers should guard against such practices by visiting an ophthalmologist and having their eyes and prescription checked regularly.

Finding an Ophthalmologist

If you do not have a regular ophthalmologist and wonder how to find a good one, ask your family doctor to recommend one to you. If you happen to be located within a reasonable distance of a teaching hospital, call the department of ophthalmology there and ask for the name of one or more staff ophthalmologists who have private practices in your area. A third possibility is to call or write the national headquarters of the American Academy of Ophthalmology (see appendix), and ask them to send you a directory of member doctors in your area. Almost all members of this national academic organization have been granted board certification in the specialty of ophthalmology. Although neither board certification nor affiliation with a teaching hospital is an absolute guarantee of quality, both are good indications of professional expertise, so you should emphasize these two criteria in your search.

Other sources of information available at most local libraries are directories of medical specialists published by the American Board of Medical Specialists and Marquis Who's Who, which list all board-certified specialists, including ophthalmologists, and indicate their medical training and hospital affiliation.

If you have the name of an ophthalmologist, a call to a

toll-free telephone number, 1-800-776-CERT, will tell you if he or she is board certified, and if so, the year in which the certification took effect. This service will not provide you with names.

When you call to make an appointment with an ophthalmologist you have chosen, make certain to ask the receptionist about the fee schedule. Useful and acceptable questions focus on the fees for an initial complete medical eye examination and a return complete medical eye checkup. Fees obviously vary from area to area. Do not hesitate to shop around if you are quoted fees that seem too expensive for your specific locality.

When you make your first visit, feel free to decide for yourself whether or not you feel comfortable with that particular eye doctor. Medical expertise is certainly a major quality to look for in a doctor, but a good rapport and a feeling of trust are equally important, and you should not be treated by a doctor you do not like.

Specialist or Generalist?

There is an increasing trend in ophthalmology toward subspecialization. Some doctors are retinal specialists, others glaucoma specialists. Many people find this confusing and wonder how they can be sure they have found the right kind of ophthalmologist if they do not know what their problem is to begin with—or even if they have any problem at all. In general, if you have no known eye problem, the best bet is to see a general ophthalmologist. If a medical problem shows up, chances are the general ophthalmologist will have the experience to deal with it. If not, he or she will refer you to another doctor with experience in the disease you have or type of surgery you need.

Eye Medications:
Over-the-Counter and Prescription Products

Pharmaceutical and personal-care manufacturers have developed an enormous variety of over-the-counter products for consumers to put in and around their eyes. Most produce no benefit to eye health, comfort, or appearance. Used according to directions, they will do no harm, but they are of little or no good.

This may come as a surprise to those who feel that eyedrops, eyewashes, or vitamin supplements must be helpful to the eyes in some way. The fact is that nature has provided eyes with their own protective and maintenance systems, and no additional help is necessary. Tears and the blinking reflex lubricate and clean the eyes constantly.

Red Eyes

Many people are concerned about red eyes, probably because a great deal of advertising implies that redness of the eyes is a common and significant problem. The fact is that we all have small blood vessels in the membrane that covers the white of our eyes. In some people these vessels are more pronounced than in others, making their eyes look redder. This is an anatomical variation, not an indication of any sort of disorder or eye-health problem. Eyes can also become redder than normal as a result of smoking, keeping late hours, exposure to air pollutants, heavy drinking, or long, strenuous use. But despite some discomfort and an appearance you might not find pleasing, there is nothing basically wrong with red eyes.

No over-the-counter medicines are ever needed for this condition. Either you do not need any medication at all for your eyes or you have a medical eye problem, in which case you need your doctor's advice and a prescription.

If you feel you want to use eyedrops or an eyewash for their soothing effect, the best are those referred to as *artificial tears*—thickened synthetic versions of natural tears. They are nonmedical, available without a prescription, and completely harmless. They are not the same as the popular patent eye preparations that claim to reduce redness. These eyedrops contain very weak decongestants, which constrict the eye blood vessels slightly for a few minutes, long enough for you to inspect your eyes in the mirror. A short while after that, the effect has vanished. These antiredness drops are worse than useless—they are a waste of money.

A popular home remedy for tired, red eyes is a compress made from wet tea bags or slices of cucumber. This may appeal to those who like "natural" approaches to health, but they are no more or less effective than anything else. You will certainly not injure your eyes with tea bags or cucumbers, but they will not benefit your eyes either.

Certainly the most economical way to soothe the eyes is with plain water. Applying a cool compress or even rinsing the eyes with cool water from the faucet will do as much as those eye preparations sold in the drugstore. Water cannot harm the eyes, and if you find it effective for temporary relief of itchy or irritated eyes, feel free to use it.

Eye-soothing creams and line improvers are a matter of personal choice—how much they soothe and banish lines is in the eye of the beholder. Care should be taken to keep them out the eyes because they contain ingredients that may be irritating.

The notion that taking vitamins, particularly vitamin A, will somehow help the eyes is a foolish one. If you eat even a reasonably adequate diet, you are getting all the vitamins your eyes can possibly use. Do not waste your money on vitamins for your eyes.

Money-Saving Strategies

Whether you are buying nonprescription or prescription eye preparations, many are available as generics or store brands. Once the patent period for a particular drug or other product has expired, other manufacturers are free to market their own version. This permits the availability of generic preparations, which can be substantially less expensive than the name brand. These are still regulated by the Food and Drug Administration (FDA), so it is reasonable to expect them to be safe.

Today most eyedrops come prepackaged in plastic bottles with applicator tips—the eyedropper seems to have had its day. Most applicator-tip packages are sold under brand names, which may make it difficult to buy the product under its generic name. Ask your doctor to indicate the generic name so that if it is available as such, you can save what might be a considerable amount of money. In most cases, however, you will be unable to find liquid eye medications in this more economical form. Tablet and capsule drugs, which are also prescribed for eye problems, are more widely available under their generic names.

You need not be concerned about the quality of prepackaged products, but remember that prescription drugs prepared by a licensed pharmacist are not superior to those of discount pharmacies. The quality is similar and the discount price often significantly lower, so be sure to shop around for the cheapest source. The cheapest may well be a mail-order pharmacy, which is becoming a more common option especially for glaucoma patients, who have an ongoing need for eye medication. One of the most reasonable and convenient of these is a national, nonprofit mail-order service operated on a state-by-state basis by the American Association of Retired Persons (AARP). Anyone over age 50 can join AARP for a nominal annual membership fee (about $5). Members mail their prescription themselves or have their doctor phone it in to an 800 number. The medication generally arrives, postage-paid, within three days or so.

Patients who take eye medications regularly should ask their doctor to order 10 refills when the doctor writes or phones in the initial prescription. From then on, the patient can simply call the 800 number to request refills.

This and other mail-order pharmacies also carry many nonprescription items: eye preparations, contact lens solutions, and beauty and bath products, often at big discounts.

In some rural areas ophthalmologists may have dispensing facilities where they practice. This is a good idea only if no alternative source is available within a reasonable distance. Otherwise, one would have to question why an ophthalmologist would have a direct sales affiliation with a supplier of optical medical products or pharmaceuticals.

How to Administer Eye Medications

Many people find eyedrops and ointments that their doctor has prescribed much more difficult and frightening to administer than pills or ointments designed for other parts of the body. Although you may prefer to have someone else administer eye medicines, it is really quite simple to do it yourself. Here is the easiest method:

Stand in front of a mirror in good light. Do not try to put

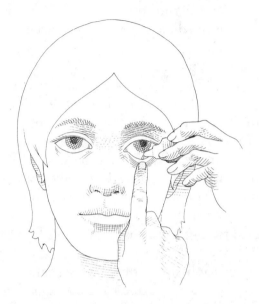

Fig. 10.4   The proper way to put in eyedrops

in eyedrops while standing over a mirror that lies flat on a table. And do not try to administer drops lying down. This "bombs away!" procedure rarely results in a direct hit. Work on one eye at a time, pulling down the lower eyelid with the fleshy pad of your index or middle finger (not with the tip or nail). Bring the dropper or dropper bottle to the eye with the other hand and squeeze gently, so a drop lands in the cul-de-sac (inside of the lower eyelid) you have exposed. Be careful not to touch the dropper tip to your eye. Release the lid. Tears and the blinking mechanism will spread the medication over the entire eyeball.

If you are not sure you got the eyedrop into your eye, put in a second one. Any excess will run out, so you are not harming the eye by putting in more. But even if you made a direct hit, some of the liquid will run out of your eye. This does *not* mean you did not get enough medication into your eye.

Use the same procedure for applying eye ointments. In this case, simply squeeze about a quarter of an inch of the medication into the bottom of the cul-de-sac and close your eyes. And again, make sure the tip of the tube does not come into contact with your eye.

Eye ointments leave a slight film over the eye that interferes somewhat with vision. Their advantage is that they work longer than drops do. For this reason, when necessary, many ophthalmologists prescribe medication in ointment form for nighttime use and in eyedrop form for use during the day.

If your doctor has prescribed two separate eyedrops, you can apply them at the same time. Wait a minute or two between applications, simply to make sure the first drops have been distributed by your tears and your blinking mechanism. It is not necessary to wait an hour or more between drops.

Most eyedrops will burn slightly in the first few moments after application because of chemical preservatives that have been added to keep the drops stable and sterile. Wait a few moments, do not rub, close your eye if that is more comfortable, and you will find that the sting quickly subsides.

If a doctor has prescribed eye medication for an infection or other acute problem (not including glaucoma medication, which must be taken regularly), discard any droppers, tubes, or other containers that remain after the condition has cleared up. Do not be tempted to save some in case the problem arises again. The preparation may have become contaminated, and a doctor should take a look at any eye that has recurrent infections or other problems.

By the same token, never let someone else use eye medication prescribed for you. The chance of spreading infection is enormous, and self-prescription or prescription by a nonmedical person is a gross violation of common sense and health safety.

Eye Cosmetics

Because our eyes are among the most physically expressive and psychologically important parts of our bodies, we should feel as good about them as we possibly can. If this includes wearing eye cosmetics, there is no reason not to do so. There is nothing inherently harmful in using eye makeup, but there are safe and unsafe ways to use it.

Always discard eye cosmetics after a few months, and never use anyone else's. Some people have allergic reactions to eye cosmetics. If you are one of these, investigate the various lines that advertise themselves as hypoallergenic. Of course, any given individual could have an allergic reaction even to these products, because none can claim to be 100 percent free of allergy-causing ingredients. Buy a small amount of one or, better yet, get a free sample if available and give it a try. If you do have an allergic response, discontinue using the cosmetic immediately. In all likelihood, the reaction will subside within a day or two.

The safe way to apply cosmetics avoids irritating the eyes. The object is to keep the cosmetics out of the eye itself. For example, when you apply mascara, do so on the outer two-thirds of the lashes only. Do not begin at the

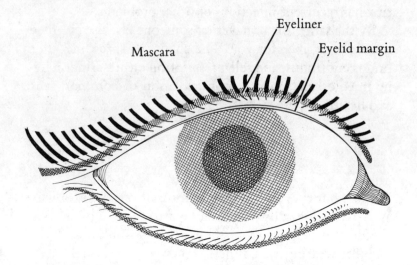

Fig. 10.5   **The safe way to apply eye makeup:**
Apply mascara to only the outer two-thirds of
the eyelashes. Apply eyeliner outside the lash
line, keeping it away from the eyelid margin.

roots, because the mascara can run into the eye or, once it
has dried, flake off and fall. Take care also when applying
eyeliner, whether the liquid or pencil/crayon type. Never
apply liner to the inner eyelid margins. Instead, put it on
just above the eyelashes of the upper lid and just below the
eyelashes of the lower lid. This may mean revising your eye
makeup design; it also will keep you from lining your eyes
instead of your eyelids and ending up with major eye complaints. Keeping just to the outside of the lashes will minimize the chance of poking the pencil or applicator in your
eye and having the liner run or flake off into your eye.

Apply eyeliner gently, being careful not to bear down hard on the eylid. Take care not to poke a pencil or applicator into your eye. If you use the crayon-type liner, warm the point for a moment with your fingertips to soften it. This will make application easier and smoother.

Eye shadow or other creams intended for the eyelids should also be kept out of the eyes. Begin a small distance away from the margins, and apply gently.

False eyelashes warrant caution. Regardless of the type you use, you will be working with glue. Be extremely careful not to get any of this in your eyes, and discontinue using it if you have an allergic reaction to the adhesive.

The so-called permanent false eyelashes, which can be left on for several months, are another matter. There is a danger that these will block the normal secretions of the eyelid glands and result in infection—sties and chalazions in particular. At least with the sort of eyelash that is removed each night, it is possible to clean the eyelids and permit gland secretion to proceed normally during sleep.

Another cosmetic treatment that can be hazardous is eyelash curling. If you must curl your lashes, begin away from the edge of the eyelids so you do not pinch the sensitive skin. Do not pull or twist the curler once the eyelashes are clamped into it. Other than that, you are on your own if curly lashes are your idea.

How you remove eye makeup is a matter of personal preference. You can wash with soap and water or apply a cleansing cream or oil, or use one of the premoistened, oily pads advertised especially for makeup removal. Whichever method you choose, keep your eyes closed, take care not to let any makeup or remover run into your eyes, and do not bear down hard or rub. The gentlest touch should do the job and avoid irritation of your eyes.

Contact lens wearers should put in their lenses after applying eye makeup and remove them before removing makeup.

Eyestrain

There is a collection of symptoms that both doctors and patients lump under the term *eyestrain,* which includes tiring of the eyes when reading, a tight or pulling sensation around the brows, and a general feeling of fatigue centered in the eyes. Although the cause can certainly be some sort of eye-muscle imbalance or may indicate a need for glasses, frequently an individual has simply reached his or her threshold of eye use and is ready for a rest. An eye doctor can rule out muscle imbalance or the need for glasses, or if one of these is the cause, can treat the problem.

Eyestrain is frustrating, but it is important to realize that eyes have limits. If you run around the block for 20 minutes and your legs get tired, this does not mean there is something wrong with your legs and you need crutches; it simply means that you should take a short rest before running again. Your neighbor may be able to run for 40 minutes without tiring, and your spouse may be able to manage only 10. The point at which eyes get tired is also an individual matter. By and large we must live with these differences, but there are some commonsense measures to maximize the amount of time you can read or use your eyes intensely before tiring. Inadequate sleep, tension, poor diet, and poor general health all contribute to eye fatigue. Take care of yourself, mind and body, and you will probably experience less eyestrain.

And when you do feel your eyes getting tired, take a

break. Close your eyes for a few minutes or gaze out the window or even at the ceiling. After this rest you will be able to resume reading with greater comfort.

Proper Lighting

Many people consider proper lighting to be an essential element in preventive eye care. Mothers have been haranguing children for decades, if not centuries, not to read in poor light. Their intentions are admirable, but the fact is that you cannot harm your eyes by reading or doing any kind of seeing in less than "good" light.

This does not mean you should read in the dark. There is a proper level and location of light for reading that will help you see better and cut down on eyestrain. But this is a matter of comfort, not medical eye health.

The best light setup for reading has the light source located behind you—it can be behind one or both shoulders—and is directed onto the page. In this way, what you are looking at will be lighted, but you will not have light glaring into your eyes, as you would if the light source were in front of you. Within reasonable bounds, the brighter the light, the better, since it will provide more contrast and make the words on the page easier to read. Obviously, a light so bright that its glare bothers you is too bright.

The second-best setup is with a shielded light in front of you and aimed at the page. The small high-intensity halogen lamps are the most common example of such lighting. Their effect is essentially the same as the first option, because the shield keeps the light from your eyes and directs it to the page.

Choose the sort of lamp and lighting that provide the

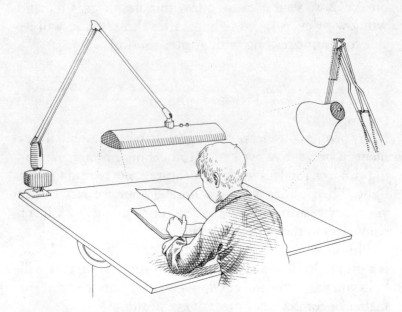

Fig. 10.6　Two proper lighting arrangements: shielded front lighting and over-the-shoulder back lighting

most comfortable light. Whether it is fluorescent or incandescent light makes no difference. Many people find fluorescent light too harsh. If you do, use an incandescent bulb. Neither is better or worse for your eyes.

It is similarly unimportant how the rest of the room is lighted. There is no advantage to a darkened room, leaving you to read in a pool of light; nor is it any better to read in a well-lighted room.

When you can control the manner and type of lighting, arrange it so it is comfortable to you. If it is beyond your control, do not worry about injuring your eyesight or eye health. You will not.

How to Buy a Pair of Glasses

If your eye doctor prescribes glasses, the next step is up to you. Ophthalmologists do not make glasses; glasses must be ordered through an *optician,* a specially trained and licensed technician who dispenses lenses according to prescription.

If you do not know where to go for your glasses, you can ask your eye doctor to recommend a particular optician. If the doctor does not wish to recommend an optician, or if you prefer to find one on your own, the best bet is usually the neighborhood optician, who has a single shop. This is preferable to visiting a franchise or an outfit that is part of a large chain. If the neighborhood optician has a good reputation among people you know, you should feel confident about buying your eyeglasses there.

The great majority of states require opticians to be licensed. The quality of workmanship in grinding and dispensing lenses is most important where greater optical errors are involved, when certain eye-muscle problems are present, or when the patient knows he or she has a complicated prescription.

Discount optical houses are a less desirable choice. They are often chains. They frequently advertise on television, radio, and in newspapers, offering huge selections of fashion frames and fast, often same-day service. They depend on volume sales, and their work tends to be sloppy. The frames and lenses they sell are usually not of the same high quality as those available through neighborhood opticians, and high-pressure selling often goes along with the promises of low price and high fashion. Furthermore, the salesperson who fits glasses at these outlets is most likely not an optician at all but simply a clerk.

Glasses are also made by optometrists, who are qualified to test eyes for nonmedical defects of vision. If you have had your eyes examined by an optometrist, he or she will make your glasses. If an ophthalmologist has written your prescription, you can also have the glasses made by an optometrist recommended by the ophthalmologist or by other customers you know. Again, a neighborhood establishment rather than a chain is the wisest choice.

Purchasing glasses is a serious matter requiring careful consideration and expert, objective advice. Glasses must serve your daily visual needs, and you must feel comfortable with the appearance and fit of both lens and frame. Because glasses are an expensive investment, it is important to make the purchase calmly, carefully, and without being subjected to pressure. This is often difficult at the discount houses. Wherever you purchase your glasses, make certain *you* are satisfied—with the glasses themselves and with the price you are paying. Take your time and do not allow yourself to be rushed. Take along a friend if you feel you need a second opinion on how the frames look. This is particularly valuable if you see so badly without your glasses that you cannot tell how you look in a particular pair of frames.

A common experience for shoppers at discount optical shops is that they are talked into buying additional pairs of glasses that they do not need. If you require more than one pair of glasses, your eye doctor will discuss this with you and give you a prescription for each. Do not be badgered into buying additional glasses. The only case in which you might want an additional pair is if you have decided to purchase sunglasses. Discuss this with your doctor and get a prescription that suits your outdoor viewing needs.

If you find yourself being pressured by an optician, leave the store. The optician should return your prescription to you on your request, but if this is awkward, simply ask your eye doctor to send you another one or have your new optician telephone for it. Similarly, if you are confused in any way by the advice of an optician—or about any other matter regarding the purchase of glasses—do not hesitate to call your eye doctor before proceeding with your purchase. It is also a good idea to find out what the total cost of your glasses will be before ordering them. If a new pair of glasses does not feel comfortable, allow a few days to get used to a new prescription. If you are still uncomfortable after that, go back and ask the optician to check that the prescription was correctly made and the glasses properly centered. If everything is as it should be but the glasses still do not feel right, have your eye doctor recheck the prescription.

Aside from opticians and optometrists, some reading glasses can be purchased in drug and variety stores and by mail. These ready-made reading glasses are an acceptable, cheap alternative for people who have no optical error other than presbyopia, for which they need magnifying glasses when reading and doing close work. They are available in .25-diopter increments, from +1.00 diopter (the weakest) to +3.50 diopters (the strongest) strength. The magnification is always the same for both eyes. If an opthalmologist has given you a clean bill of health after a complete medical eye check, and if you find these glasses comfortable and can find a style that pleases you, there is no reason to spend more on custom-made glasses.

Lens Materials

Although by custom they are still called eyeglasses, it is the rare corrective lens in the United States today that is actually made of glass. Plastic is lighter, can be made resistant to scratching, and is shatterproof. FDA regulations require glass lenses to be impact-resistant, which is accomplished by heat or chemical treatment, but it results in a thicker lens.

The type of plastic influences the final cost. Hyperindex 160 plastic has a cosmetic advantage by permitting thinner edges and thus an overall thinner appearance. This may be worth the expense to people with relatively serious nearsightedness or farsightedness, which requires a fairly thick lens. Hyperindex 160 comes with ultraviolet-screen and scratchguard coating, and costs about double that of lenses made from standard plastic.

Polycarbon is another special plastic used in making lenses. The advantage here is strength: This material is used for bulletproof shields. Glasses made of polycarbon may be of value to children, athletes, or those with certain occupational needs. A very sharp or high-velocity object could pierce a regular plastic lens, but would be repelled by a polycarbon lens. Polycarbon does not tint well, 33 percent being the maximum tint obtainable. The cost again is about double, and UV coating and scratchguard are included.

These two options and several others are available at extra cost on other types of plastic lenses. Ultraviolet coating, which screens out rays from the sun that are thought to contribute to cataract formation, adds about 20 percent to the cost of regular plastic lenses. The coating is invisible and should not be confused with tinting used for sunglasses. There is no need to protect the eyes from ultraviolet radiation indoors, so the additional cost is probably not worth it for anyone who will be wearing separate sunglasses outdoors.

Another option is glare-free coating, which renders the lenses essentially invisible to anyone looking at the wearer.

A lens so treated would, for example, not reflect glare in a photograph. It does not, however, protect the wearer from glare, making the additional 50 percent charge a dubious expenditure for those other than models and celebrities who wear glasses in front of the camera.

Tinting increases the cost of lenses by about 20 percent. It can be done at the time the glasses are originally made up or it can be added later. Tints can range from 5 percent, for an added color that is cosmetic only, to 92 percent, for highly protective sunglasses.

Sunglasses

Sunglasses are heavily tinted glasses meant to be worn outdoors as protection from the sun's glare. They can be made up with or without optical correction. There are various intensities and various colors available in sunglasses, and which you select is a matter of personal preference. No particular color has any medical superiority over another, nor can any color per se be harmful to the eyes. It is a good idea to shop for sunglasses on a sunny day; that way, you can test the various intensities and colors outdoors and select the one most comfortable for you.

Unlike clear glasses worn indoors, sunglasses should have an ultraviolet coating. The tint filters *visible* light; it is the *invisible*, ultraviolet light that causes skin cancer and may hasten the development of cataracts. Many sunglasses, prescription and otherwise, are available with UV coating. Caveat emptor, however, when buying from a source other than a reputable optician: Just because a lens carries a sticker saying it protects against ultraviolet rays does not make it so. Although a sunglass industry group has devised standards for UV filtration, no government agency oversees this and there is nothing to prevent a vendor from affixing a sticker to any pair of sunglasses, whether the lenses are specially coated or not.

As far as color goes, gray is probably the best choice because it is a neutral tint, which minimizes color distortion. Also, the maximum dark gray is the darkest tint possible, permitting only 10 percent light transmission. Green or brown cannot be made quite as dark, and they distort color more. Light colors such as pink or yellow are purely cosmetic as they do not exclude enough light to have a practical effect.

Sunglasses with gradient lenses—dark at the top and gradually lightening until they are almost clear at the bottom—are of no optical or medical benefit. The choice of these glasses is a matter of fashion and taste, but do test them out in sunlight before buying, since they may not provide sufficient protection against glare to suit your needs.

The most economical way to get the benefits of prescription sunglasses is to buy a pair of tinted clip-ons. Available in drugstores and variety stores at reasonable prices, these sunshields do not, of course, contain any prescription, but because they can be attached to regular glasses, they provide protection against bright sunlight while your own glasses provide the optical correction.

If you are in the market for nonprescription sunglasses, you need not be afraid of ruining your eyes with a cheap pair. A more expensive pair is a better buy simply because sturdier frames will probably last longer and fit better, and a better optical-quality lens will give less distortion. Sunglasses are rarely a matter of medical necessity, but if you feel the personal need for them, by all means invest in a pair.

Other Issues When Choosing Glasses

The two factors that go into the choice of a frame are sturdiness and fashion. It is probably worth paying more for a sturdier frame; whether one wishes to pay more to make a fashion statement is an individual matter. Frame size is also a question of personal preference. There is nothing wrong with wearing large glasses if you like the way you look in them, but they are usually more expensive, and in the outer reaches of the lens the distortion tends to be quite pronounced. Do not expect to be able to look far out to the side or down in the corner of an oversized lens and see a clear, focused image—it is simply too far from the optical center of the lens.

In choosing frames, metal or plastic, colored or plain, size and shape are all questions to be answered. Another is whether or not you want to pay the considerable added expense of a new type of frame made from a titanium alloy, which will spring back to its original shape even if you sit on it. These frames do not crack, break, or lose their original contours.

With sunglasses, a large frame or even a wraparound-style frame may be desirable because they protect more of the area around the eyes from sun damage.

Some Tips on Eyeglass Care and Maintenance

Once you have your glasses, a certain amount of care is required so they will continue to provide good visual correction.

The most obvious point is to keep the glasses clean. Oil from your skin and dust and grit in the air will cling to the

lenses. Clean them off whenever they need it, but certainly
at least once a day. The best way to do this is with a clean,
soft cloth or one of the special lens-cleaning papers available at drugstores and optical stores. Some opticians recommend that glasses, especially plastic ones, be cleaned
when wet, in order to reduce the chance of scratching. You
can use special lens-cleaning fluids, or plain tap water with
or without a bit of soap.

It is also a good idea to keep your glasses in a case when
you are not using them, particularly if you are carrying
them in a purse or in your pocket. The case will keep the
frames from getting bent, protect the glasses if they are
dropped, and keep the lenses from getting scratched. If you
take off your glasses at home and do not put them in a case,
lay them on their sides so they rest on the frame. Never
place them lens side down.

If your lenses do become scratched enough to interfere
with vision, nothing can be done if they are plastic lenses.
However, glass lenses can sometimes be repolished and
recoated. This works only if the scratches are not too deep,
but it is a possible remedy.

Ill-fitting or loose frames that slide down your nose or sit
askew on your face will not allow you to get the best benefits of your prescription, because the optical center of the
lens must be directly in front of the pupil. This is why a
careful and conscientious optician will spend what may
seem like an excessive amount of time adjusting your
frames. If you drop your glasses, if the screws in the hinges
become loose, of if the frames get bent, have them read-
justed and repaired so alignment is again perfect. And if you
have wire frames, you should have the alignment checked
periodically. This type is particularly prone to bending. Do
not continue to wear glasses that are askew, and do not

attempt to repair them yourself with paper clips or bits of wire. In most cases, the optician from whom you bought your glasses will make these repairs and adjustments free, but in any case the charge will be nominal and definitely worth it.

People who are very dependent on their glasses should keep an extra pair on hand. This is obviously a good thing if you lose your glasses and have to wait a few days to get a new pair made. Most economical is to save your last pair of glasses, which will be adequate for a short time. If you want to spend the money, you can certainly buy two pairs of glasses with your current prescription, but this is not really

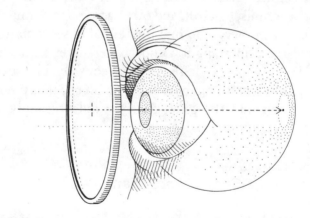

Fig. 10.7   The optical center of an eyeglass lens, the only
            point of perfect correction, should sit directly
            in front of the center of the pupil.

necessary. It also might be a good idea to keep a copy of your prescription, especially if you are traveling. The "language" of eyeglass prescriptions is universal; opticians from Paris to Hong Kong can make a new pair of glasses as quickly and easily as can their counterparts in your hometown.

Special Needs

Eyeglasses and physical sports are not terribly compatible. Very active people whose eyes require correction may find contact lenses better suited to their needs. Those who prefer to wear glasses should take a number of precautions. Polycarbon lenses may be worth the additional expense. Elastic eyeglass holders that fasten around the back of the head keep the glasses from falling off, and many people who play tennis, baseball, and other active sports find these helpful. Swimmers who find it essential to see well (this is particularly important for underwater divers) may wear goggles over their glasses. For a considerable sum of money, a face mask can be made with an eyeglass prescription ground into the glass. Skiers should certainly wear goggles over their glasses.

Contact Lens Economics

Where you buy your contact lenses makes a difference from an economic and medical point of view, and in this instance medical considerations should win out. Although it may be costlier to go to an ophthalmologist, you will probably get a better fit and will certainly be taking better care of the health of your eyes. Only an ophthalmologist can accurately diagnose and treat eye problems that might interfere with or result from wearing contact lenses. These include corneal abrasions, which require medical treatment.

When shopping around for an ophthalmologist to fit you with contact lenses, be sure to ask what the fee schedule is for both soft and rigid gas-permeable lenses. Also inquire about the fitting, the lenses themselves, and the follow-up visits. If you already have an ophthalmologist, these questions are equally valid. Even though the prices quoted probably will be higher than the special deals offered by many optical chains, the security that you are not putting the health of your eyes in jeopardy should be worth the additional cost.

Lens Solutions

The cleaning and storage solutions for contact lenses represent one class of nonprescription eye products that is necessary, and can represent a significant expense. But even in this group, some are required for hygienic maintenance of the lenses and others are just frills. Much depends on the type of lenses you wear. Many of these products are available as generics or store brands; when available from a mail-order pharmacy, they may also be found at reduced prices.

Soft-Lens Solutions

Because they are made from a highly absorbent gel, soft lenses must be kept wet and must be sterilized periodically to avoid bacterial contamination. The most economical way to ensure this is with the old-fashioned heat cleaner as well as normal saline (salt solution). Normal saline can be obtained by mixing a salt tablet and distilled water. (Do *not* use table salt and tap water!) Prepackaged cleaning and soaking solutions and normal saline without preservatives cost more, but many people judge the convenience worth the additional price.

Enzyme tablets to loosen protein deposits are necessary only for those who tend to build up excessive protein in their soft lenses. An ophthalmologist should advise on this.

Rigid-Lens Solutions

Prepackaged cleaning and soaking solutions are the only choice for gas-permeable and hard contact lenses. Buy the type designed for the lenses you have. Many contain preservatives, which may irritate the eyes. If so, try a different brand or one without a preservative, in which case you must watch the expiration date carefully. If you find you are discarding a lot of solution after the time expires, buy smaller quantities.

Contact Lens Insurance

Contact lens insurance is generally available from contact lens providers only, who may urge or otherwise pressure wearers to purchase their insurance. Some providers do not even offer this service because they feel it is a poor bargain for the consumer as well as poor use of their own office time. Unless you are a contact lens loser or quite careless about lens maintenance, insurance is probably not economical. Ask your provider the cost of a replacement lens without insurance, under what conditions the particular policy being offered will cover replacement, and what the per-

claim deductibles and annual premiums are. *Be independent.*
Use the answers to make your own decision whether or not
insurance makes sense for you. It is generally true that the
replacement cost is not much higher than the deductible;
adding the premium, the consumer would usually have to
replace two lenses a year to gain a net profit sufficient to
cover the mailing costs and aggravation.

Visual Training for Learning Problems

Referring schoolchildren to visual training centers is a
recent trend that has unfortunately become a national
mania. Well-meaning but misinformed teachers and others
attribute reading and learning difficulties to eye problems
that can be solved by so-called visual training.

These learning problems usually crop up in grade school,
after the visual learning period has ended. They must be
distinguished from the normal tendency of children when
learning to read and write to reverse or even invert numbers
and letters. This experimental phase passes quickly as children become more familiar with these new symbols and
correct themselves. It is analogous to the first tentative steps
and tumbles taken by a child learning to walk.

The so-called visual training centers, which are staffed
exclusively by optometrists and nonmedical technicians,
can do absolutely nothing to correct the so-called problem
or hasten learning to read and write. Glowing reports from
parents whose children have had visual training are invariably the result of the fact that the training coincided with
the period when the child would, as a matter of course,
have begun to write properly. In this way, this expensive

and time-consuming process feeds on itself, garnering credit that properly belongs to the passage of time rather than to any virtue of the program.

This is not to say that there is no such thing as a learning disability. Optical defects or neurological or psychological problems can cause a child to have a difficult time in school, but these are matters for diagnosis and treatment by eye doctors, neurologists, or psychiatrists. An ophthalmologist can tell by examining a child's eyes whether the problem is a real one requiring optical or surgical correction, if the child is simply going through the normal period of visual orientation, or if, in the absence of any eye problem, consultation with a neurologist or psychiatrist is recommended.

Health Insurance

Health insurance is of enormous value for the maintenance of eye health. People with glaucoma, who must have frequent checks of their intraocular pressure, avoid much of the financial burden of these office visits if they have adequate medical insurance. Cataract surgery is a very expensive proposition for anyone not well covered, but even people who have no eye disease and are simply following the judicious course of having annual medical eye checkups can benefit from health insurance. It can often make that office visit cheaper than a visit to an optometrist.

Private Insurance

Although most private policies will not pay for preventive care, a medical eye examination often yields a diagnosis of some sort and that justifies reimbursement for the visit. For example, you may have some symptoms you wish the doctor to investigate in the course of the examination. And even if you have no specific complaint, there is still a very high probability that your eyes, although healthy, have some abnormality, even a minor one. This would permit the ophthalmologist to make a diagnosis.

If you have private coverage, make certain you have a paid receipt, plus a bill with a diagnosis, for reimbursement. Most doctors will submit both receipt and bill for you, or provide you with a combination receipt/report that need only be attached to the insurance form for submission. If you are intimidated by the reimbursement procedure, look for an eye doctor whose office is willing to submit insurance forms for patients.

HMOs

An increasingly common alternative to health insurance, the Health Maintenance Organization (HMO), does pay for preventive care. Subscribers prepay an annual fee in exchange for medical care, including routine checkups. Rather than choosing private doctors, subscribers generally are given a choice among member physicians. Most have ophthalmologists and optometrists on their staffs, and some even have member opticians.

As health cost pressures increase, corporations are looking on HMOs with increasing favor as a way to curb employee health-care costs. Some HMOs are old, well-established, and economically stable. Some of the newer ones may be economically unstable or even in debt. Before choosing to join an HMO, consumers are well advised to scrutinize its history and its financial status carefully. It is often helpful to ask other people you know what their experience has been with a given HMO. Find out in advance whether you will have a choice of doctors, and whether you will always see the same doctor. Inquire about eligible services for eye care, glasses, contact lenses, and eye surgery.

Medicare

If you are over 65 or disabled and you have Part B Medicare (the optional doctor coverage, which is automatically deducted from your monthly Social Security check), 80 percent of reasonable and customary fees in your geographical area will be paid. It is a good idea to inquire in advance whether an ophthalmologist you plan to use is a Medicare participant. If so, 80 percent of the usual fee will be sent directly to the ophthalmologist and you will be billed only for the 20 percent balance. The so-called Medigap policies, private supplementary insurance for Medicare-eligible individuals, will cover the 20 percent difference.

If you want to find an ophthalmologist who accepts Medicare, a phone call to 800-222-EYES will give you a list of participating ophthalmologists in your area. Such a list is available directly from Medicare as well.

If you are eligible for Medicare but choose a doctor who is not a Medicare participant, federal law restricts the fee you can be charged. Depending on the examination or procedure, the ceiling is 15 to 40 percent in excess of the fee allowed by Medicare.

Federal law also requires that all providers, whether Medicare participants or not, submit Medicare claim forms for their eligible patients.

Getting a Second Opinion

An adjunct to medical insurance is the second opinion, a practice that can benefit patients greatly and reduce the incidence of unnecessary procedures. If for any reason you have a doubt about the diagnosis and treatment you are receiving, by all means get a second opinion. No professional who is competent and confident would have any objection to a patient seeking corroborating or even contradictory advice from another professional. If you are facing eye surgery, many insurance companies require a second opinion before they will approve payment for a surgical procedure.

Guidelines for finding a qualified ophthalmologist to give you a second opinion include board certification and affiliation with a teaching hospital, if at all possible. Another physician you know is a valid referral source, as may be friends who are patients of another ophthalmologist. Your current ophthalmologist is not.

Some Hazards of Modern Medicine to Avoid

Unnecessary Tests

Soaring malpractice insurance costs and claims in our litigious society have justifiably caused many doctors to keep one eye on their patients and the other on their lawyers. There is no doubt that defensive medicine is a reality today. One by-product of that is extensive and often excessive testing, often ordered more as protection for the doctor than to obtain information about the patient. A good relationship between patient and doctor is the best antidote: An honest discussion about how necessary an expensive test really is may result in delaying or deferring the test completely.

Consumers should be aware of a particular practice by a few ophthalmologists today that may not be motivated by concern for patient welfare. This is the use of high-tech tests in circumstances where such tests are absolutely unnecessary. What must come to mind is that they are being used to turn a profit. A prime example of this abuse is the B-scan, a completely safe, noninvasive sonar testing device that makes a picture of the eyeball and reveals various tissue densities. B-scans are beneficial in diagnosing tumors of the eye, and when indicated, they can be very useful. Needless to say, this test garners a fairly high insurance reimbursement. Coupled with its safety and ease of use, the high monetary return has led to gross overuse. It is arguable that the great majority of B-scans are unnecessary.

Sales representatives for manufacturers routinely visit ophthalmology practices in order to pitch their products. They claim that the products will pay for themselves in a short period of time, thanks to a quoted number of procedures fully reimbursed by Medicare or other insurance carriers. Alas, some few doctors yield to the temptation.

Unnecessary Surgery

From rationalizing unnecessary testing that is absolutely safe, it is a small step for a doctor to rationalize unnecessary surgery that is almost always safe. It cannot be said often enough: If you are facing surgery, get a second opinion.

It is ironic that perhaps the greatest surgical abuse in ophthalmology today is with the tool also responsible for its greatest real advance over the last two decades: the laser. For example, the laser is widely used today for retinal surgery, which is, sadly, one of the most abused and unnecessary surgical eye procedures. If an ophthalmologist tells you that you need laser treatment for a retinal hole, tear, or detachment, get a second opinion. If he or she tells you it is an emergency, *rush* to a second opinion. Laser treatment for one of these retinal problems is never a true emergency.

In glaucoma, laser surgery is a miraculous improvement over traditional intraocular surgery. When medically indicated, laser surgery represents a revolution in safety and outcome. But here again, abuse is sadly too often the case. Laser surgery is indicated only after medical treatment has failed or if a patient cannot be made to comply with medical instructions. This is the same indication that was applied to conventional surgery before lasers were available. Yet far more laser glaucoma procedures are done than knife surgery ever was. One must conclude from this fact that part of the increase is made up of unnecessary procedures. Consumers can defend themselves against this by getting second opinions, for which there is almost always time. Except in the case of acute glaucoma, laser surgery is not an emergency.

Buccaneer Surgeons and Surgical Mills

The term "buccaneer surgeon" was used over a decade ago in an ophthalmology trade journal. It aptly refers to an unfortunate trend in which some eye surgeons alter existing procedures in small ways in order to identify themselves with an allegedly improved method. Some of this designer surgery incorporates ever higher technology, at ever higher cost, often with little or no added real benefit except in profits for the surgeon and the ophthalmic equipment industry.

Along with this seems to be a rush to quicker procedures with shorter recovery stays, more flamboyant instrumentation, sometimes with little or no added real benefit, and at times even higher operative risk. If your doctor advocates a new or unusual procedure, get a second opinion.

Doctors Who Advertise

Although advertising by doctors is now legal, the ethics and necessity of doing so are still questionable. Some doctors engage the services of public relations firms to keep themselves in the public eye. Those photographs of an eye doctor in the local newspaper or interviews on local radio and TV were probably placed by a PR firm. But while the spotlight is on such doctors, the fact remains that many of the best and brightest ophthalmologists do not advertise, and the most professional do not use public relations firms.

The Media and the Medical Consumer

Finally, a word about you, the patient, and the media. Television is insatiable for cures, the latest laser application, the miraculous procedure of the future, and other medical hype. Books, magazines, and newspapers are no less eager to explore the frontiers of modern medicine and beyond. The result is a climate in which consumers hear about exotic, frequently unproven technologies. As patients, they may pressure their physicians to treat them today with tomorrow's instrumentation and medications. Do not succumb to this temptation. As exciting as medical research is, and as much promise as it holds for future generations, it remains true that the conservative approach—the least medicine possible to get the desired result—is still the best. It is the wise patient who is a well-educated consumer, but it is usually wiser still to be a conservative patient of a conservative ophthalmologist.

Glossary

◇

This glossary includes all technical and medical terms mentioned in the text. It can be used as a companion to the text when further clarification or redefinition is needed. It also includes some entries not discussed in the text. Because this book focuses on common eye problems, these entries will serve to introduce, if only briefly, some relatively rare eye conditions.

This is, by no means, a complete eye dictionary. Readers interested in further exploration will find a variety of medical lexicons and other sources in the research section of their local library. Not included here, for example, are the names of drugs currently used in eye care, nor those of dubious, outmoded, or soon-to-be outmoded therapeutic procedures.

Absolute glaucoma. *See* Glaucoma.
Accommodation. The process in which the shape of the

273

human lens adjusts for near vision so that light rays from a near external object are brought to a point of focus on the retina.

Acute glaucoma. *See* Glaucoma.

Allergic conjunctivitis. An inflammation of the conjunctiva in response to an allergy-causing substance.

Amblyopia. A failure of normal visual development in an eye with no pathological defect and with the anatomical potential for normal vision.

Ametropia. Optical error, or a condition in which faulty refraction of light rays prevents an image from being brought to focus on the retina, as in the case of myopia, hyperopia, or astigmatism.

Aneurysm. An outpouching or enlargement of an artery that can rupture and result in a hemorrhage.

Anisocoria. Any inequality in the size of the pupils. This can be a normal anatomical variation or a sign of pathology.

Anisometropia. A condition in which the optics of one eye differ greatly from those of the other eye.

Anterior chamber. The space behind the cornea and in front of the iris that is filled with aqueous fluid.

Anterior drainage angle. The area in the anterior chamber at the junction of the cornea and iris at which the aqueous fluid drains from the eye.

Applanation tonometry. A diagnostic test for glaucoma that involves flattening the cornea by applying pressure to it as a means of measuring intraocular pressure.

Aqueous fluid. Also called aqueous humor; the watery fluid that fills the anterior and posterior chambers of the eye. It acts to nourish and lubricate the lens and cornea as well as to maintain the eyeball's consistency.

Arcus senilis. An opaque, grayish ring at the edge of the cornea that frequently occurs in older people and is the result of fatty deposits in the cornea. It has no effect on vision.

Arteriosclerosis. A disease of the circulatory system occurring primarily in the elderly. It is characterized by an inelasticity and thickening of the walls of the arteries, which in turn cause decreased flow of blood. Arteriosclerosis can be diagnosed on examination of the retinal blood vessels. It is commonly known as hardening of the arteries.

Artificial tears. A nonmedicinal, nonprescription eyedrop that acts as a lubricant and is analogous to thickened natural tear fluid.

A-scan. An instrument employing a probe applied to the cornea in order to obtain precise measure of the axial length of the eye. It is used to calculate the optical power needed for an intraocular lens implant.

Astigmatism. An optical error characterized by an unequal curvature in one or more of the eye's refractive surfaces (most commonly the cornea), and causing an object to come to focus at two points on the visual axis instead of at one point.

Bell's palsy. A peripheral facial paralysis causing the muscles on one side of the face to be completely or partially paralyzed and, thereby, interfering with normal blinking of the eye.

Bifocal age group. Refers to that group of individuals of a certain age (usually mid-40s and onward) when reading glasses are needed to correct presbyopia, and, in the presence of another optical error, a second correction is required for distance vision.

Bifocal contact lens. A type of contact lens with two separate optical corrections, one for distance vision and the other for near vision.

Bifocal lens. An optical lens having two segments, one for near vision and one for distance vision.

Binocular vision. Vision achieved when both eyes function together. This is one of the components of normal vision.

Biomicroscope. Also known as a slit lamp, an optical instrument that isolates enlarged and illuminated sections of certain anatomical structures in the eye by utilizing a thin beam of light. It is particularly useful in examining the anterior anatomy of the eye as well as the optical media.

Bitoric lens. A contact lens in which both meridians are curved, but not to the same degree, on both internal and external surfaces of the lens. It is designed to correct severe astigmatism.

Blepharitis. A noncontagious infection of the eyelid margin, particularly around the lash area.

Blind spot. The small area on the retina at which the optic nerve is attached to the eye. Because it contains no retinal tissue, it is insensitive to light, resulting in a small area of normal visual loss.

Bony orbit. The eye socket, a cavity composed of parts of seven bones and containing the eyeball, its surrounding muscles, arteries, veins, nerves, and surrounding supporting tissue.

B-scan. A diagnostic instrument using sonar technology to yield images of various densities within the eyeball. It is useful for diagnosing eye tumors.

Cataract. A loss of transparency, of any degree and for any reason, in the lens of the eye.

Cataract surgery. The surgical procedure in which a cataractous lens of the eye is removed.

Chalazion. A cystlike growth near the border of the eyelid that results from an inflammation of a gland at the eyelid margin.

Chemical conjunctivitis. An inflammation of the conjunctiva caused by contact with or fumes of chemicals or toxins. It is also known as toxic conjunctivitis.

Chlamydia. A bacterial organism, principally transmitted through sexual contact, that can infect the external eye, most commonly the cornea.

Chorioretinitis. Any inflammation of the choroid and retinal layers of the eye, usually caused by an infection elsewhere in the body.

Choroid. A delicate membranous layer of the eye that lies between the sclera and the retina and is continuous with the iris and the ciliary body in front of it. It is primarily a blood vessel layer.

Chronic simple glaucoma. *See* Glaucoma.

Cilia. The eyelashes.

Ciliary body. A vascular and muscular structure that lies between the choroid layer and the iris. It secretes aqueous fluid into the posterior chamber, and its muscles form part of the near-focusing system.

Closed angle glaucoma. *See* Glaucoma.

Cold sore. Common term for a type of blister, often seen in the mouth and nose area, and caused by the herpes simplex virus. *See also* Herpes simplex.

Color blindness. A genetically inherited birth defect that occurs almost exclusively in men and causes loss of normal color perception. The actual degree of loss varies widely.

Concave lens. A lens in which one or both surfaces are curved inward. *Compare* Convex lens.

Cones. Specialized cells of the retina sensitive to color and light intensity. They are important in light adaptation and color perception.

Congenital cataract. A rare type of cataract present at birth. *See also* Cataract.

Congenital glaucoma. *See* Glaucoma.

Conjunctiva. The mucous membrane covering the exposed front portion of the sclera and continuing to form the lining of the inside of the eyelids.

Conjunctivitis. Any inflammation of the conjunctiva and commonly known as pinkeye. *See also* Allergic conjunctivitis; Chemical conjunctivitis; Infectious conjunctivitis.

Constrictor muscles. *See* Dilator pupillae; Sphincter pupillae.

Contact lenses. A pair of small optical lenses that correct optical defects inconspicuously by resting directly on the tear layer of the cornea. They are generally made of plastic.

Convergence. The normal process in which both eyes move inward toward one another to focus on a near object.

Convergence reflex. A normal, involuntary reflex in which the visual axes of the two eyes bend toward one another as the near-focusing muscles come into use.

Convergent strabismus. *See* Esotropia.

Convex lens. A lens in which one or both surfaces are curved outward. *Compare* Concave lens.

Cornea. The curved, transparent membrane forming the front one-sixth of the outer coat of the eyeball. It serves primarily as protection and is the outermost refractive surface of the eye.

Corneal contact lenses. Contact lenses that are fitted exclusively on the corneal surface. These are the most commonly used contact lenses today.

Corneal dystrophy. Degeneration of the layers of the cornea, resulting in noninflammatory lesions that show up as clouding and cause corresponding visual loss.

Corneal transplant. A surgical procedure in which a portion of clear donor cornea is used to replace a corresponding portion of the patient's opacified cornea.

Corneal ulcer. A defect in the protective outer layer of the cornea, most commonly caused by an infection.

Cortex. Refers to the outer portion of a structure. In the human eye, it is the portion of the lens just inside the capsule and surrounding the central nucleus.

Cosmetic contact lens. A type of contact lens used to alter the color of the eyes by providing the iris with an opaque covering that resembles an iris but is of another color.

Couching. An obsolete cataract operation, it moved the lens out of the optical axis by displacing it into the vitreous fluid.

Cross-eye. A lay term for strabismus. *See* Strabismus.

Cryoextraction. A cataract removal technique employing a probe that freezes the lens, which is then removed from the eye as a single hardened unit.

Cryosurgery. Surgery involving the freezing of tissues. It is used in some cataract extractions, glaucoma operations, and retinal repairs.

Cryotherapy. The use of cold or freezing in the treatment of disease. In ophthalmology, cryotherapy is sometimes used to control glaucoma and to repair retinal tears and detachment.

Cupping of optic disc. An excavated or C-shaped portion of the optic disc. It can be a normal anatomical variation or can occur in glaucoma, in which case it may be worse.

Cyclodiathermy. The use of heat in the treatment of eye disease. As a glaucoma treatment, heat may be applied to the sclera in an attempt to lessen secretion of aqueous fluid by the ciliary body. In repair of retinal detachment, it may be applied externally to produce scar tissue adhesion between retina and choroid.

Cycloplegic drops. Dual-action diagnostic eyedrops that temporarily paralyze the near-focusing muscles of the eye as well as dilate the pupil.

Cystoid macular edema. Cystlike swelling of tissues in the central (macular) portion of the eye, resulting in visual loss. The most frequent cause is trauma, either from a blow to the eye or as a complication of intraocular surgery.

Cytomegalovirus. One of a group of herpes viruses that not infrequently infect the retina of AIDS patients.

Dacryoadenitis. Any infection of the lacrimal gland.

Dacryocystitis. Any infection of the lacrimal sac.

Dacryocystorhinostomy. A surgical procedure in which an artificial opening is created between the lacrimal sac and the nasal cavity, facilitating tear drainage when scar tissue has blocked the normal drainage pathways.

Dark adaptation. The ability of the eye to adjust itself to decreasing illumination. This process occurs in the retina and entails an increase in the number of functioning rods and a decrease in the number of functioning cones. Complete dark adaptation takes about one hour. *Compare* Light adaptation.

Dendritic ulcer. An ulcer of the cornea caused by the herpes simplex virus. It has a characteristic appearance resembling the branches of a tree.

Deviant eye. An eye that is not fixing on the object being viewed but is turned away from the visual axis. This term is used in reference to strabismus.

Diabetes, or diabetes mellitus. A metabolic disorder characterized by an imbalance in blood sugar levels in the body. It can have damaging effects on the eye as well as on the rest of the body.

Diabetic cataract. A clouding of the lens of the eye caused by diabetes. *See also* Cataract.

Diabetic retinopathy. A catchall term used to describe any of the various stages of retinal pathology caused by diabetes, including hemorrhages, thrombi, aneurysms, and scarring of the retinal tissue.

Dilator muscles. *See* Dilator pupillae; Sphincter pupillae.

Dilator pupillae. A muscle situated in the peripheral part of the iris in which contraction of the iris causes dilation of the pupil and relaxation allows the pupil to contract.

Diopter. The unit used to measure the light-bending power of a lens.

Diplopia. Double vision, a pathological condition of vision in which a single object is perceived as two.

Discission. Cutting into the capsule of the lens and breaking up the lens parts with a surgical instrument or laser beam.

Distance vision. Use of the eyes to view objects in the distance. Theoretically, that distance can be infinite. The ophthalmological measurement of distance vision is made 20 feet from the eye. In practical terms, one uses distance vision to view anything that is beyond what is considered middle distance. *See also* Middle-distance vision.

Divergence. The normal movement or spreading apart of the eyes in an outward direction.

Divergent strabismus. *See* Exotropia.

Double vision. *See* Diplopia.

Dyslexia. An inability to read with comprehension at a level indicated by the individual's overall intelligence and/or verbal skills. In medical usage, it refers to problems caused by a central (neurological) defect; in common usage, it is inaccurately used to describe any reading difficulty, such as letter inversion.

Ectropion. A condition in which the eyelid margin (usually the lower eyelid) turns outward so that the conjunctival lining is exposed.

Edema. An excessive accumulation of clear watery fluid in any tissue, resulting in the swelling of that tissue.

Embolism. The blockage of a blood vessel by a blood clot that has been carried by the bloodstream and has become impacted in some portion of the circulatory system. It often causes a secondary hemorrhage.

Emmetropia. The normal optical condition of the eye that permits rays of light to focus accurately on the retina.

Entropion. A constant or intermittent turning inward of the eyelid margin (usually the lower eyelid), causing the eyelashes to rub against the cornea. This generally occurs only in the elderly, and causes the eye to become red and irritated.

Enucleation. A surgical procedure in which the entire eyeball is removed.

Epicanthal fold. *See* Epicanthus.

Epicanthus. An anatomical feature in which a fold of skin extending from the top of the nose to the inner end of the eyebrow overlaps the inner corner of the eye. In some circumstances it can give the appearance of strabismus. It tends to recede as the bridge of the nose narrows in the course of early childhood.

Epiphora. A condition in which tears overflow onto the cheek because of a narrowing of the tear removal apparatus. Less commonly, it can result from an excessive secretion of tears.

Episcleritis. *See* Scleritis.

Esophoria. A tendency of one eye to deviate inwardly when the eyes are at rest, such as when the eyes are closed. To a small degree, this can be normal.

Esotropia. A type of strabismus in which the deviation of one eye is inward, or convergent, at rest or in use. It is also known as convergent strabismus.

Exophoria. A tendency of one eye to deviate outwardly when the eyes are at rest. To a small degree, it can be normal; to a larger degree, it can cause eye fatigue.

Exophthalmos. A forward protrusion of the eyeball, frequently caused by an overactive thyroid gland or any type of growth located in the bony orbit.

Exotropia. A type of strabismus in which the deviation of one eye is outward, or divergent, at rest or in use. It is also known as divergent strabismus.

Expulsive choroidal hemorrhage. Massive bleeding within the eye, breaking through both the choroid and retina and causing the expulsion of the contents of the eye. It is a rare complication of intraocular surgery.

Extended-wear contact lens. A contact lens designed to be worn at all times, including during sleep.

External eye muscles. *See* Extraocular muscles.

Extracapsular cataract extraction. A cataract extraction procedure in which the anterior capsule of the lens is cut and a portion removed along with the lens, but the posterior capsule is left intact. It is used in conjunction with intraocular lens implants.

Extraocular muscles. The six muscles of the eye, each of which are attached to the outside of the eyeball behind the conjunctival cul-de-sac and fastened by way of a system of connective tissue to the bony orbit. The muscles function to move the eye in its various directions to permit full 360-degree movement of the eyes, and consist of the medial rectus, lateral rectus, superior rectus, inferior rectus, superior oblique, and inferior oblique muscles.

Eye bank. A medical facility that keeps the eyes of deceased donors. The eyes are used in corneal transplantation.

Eyebrow. The crescent-shaped line of hair at the upper edge of the orbit.

Eyelid. One of the two movable folds of skin lined on the inside with conjunctival membrane and contiguous on the outside with the skin of the face. It functions to clean, lubricate, and protect the eyeball.

Eyelid tic. *See* Fibrillation.

Farsighted astigmatism. A type of astigmatism in which both points of focus have not yet been reached when light rays arrive at the retina.

Farsightedness. *See* Hyperopia.

Fibrillation. A twitching of one or both eyelids, usually the result of tension or anxiety. It is also known as eyelid tic.

Filtration procedure. A standard surgical knife procedure in the treatment of glaucoma, it results in the creation of a channel from the anterior chamber into a space under the conjunctiva through which aqueous fluid can drain.

Fixing eye. An eye that is looking straight along the visual axis at the object being viewed. This term is used in reference to strabismus.

Floaters. A common term used to describe an aggregate of cells or protein in the vitreous fluid and seen as small, moving black shapes, especially visible against a light background. This condition is usually of no pathological significance. It is also known as vitreous floaters.

Fluorescein angiography. A diagnostic procedure utilizing a special dye and photographic technique to examine the fundus of the eye.

Focal length. The distance between a refractive surface and the point at which the light rays meet.

Focus. The point at which light rays meet after passing through a refractive surface.

Focusing ability. *See* Accommodation.

Focusing muscles. A common term used to denote the anatomical system used in the process of accomodation. The system consists of the ciliary body muscles, the zonule, and the lens itself.

Fovea centralis. The small, normal anatomical depression located in the center of the macula.

Fundus. The back portion of the interior of the eyeball consisting primarily of the retina, the optic disc, and the retinal blood vessels. It can be viewed and examined with the ophthalmoscope.

Fusion. The process in which the two disparate images seen by each eye are blended into one image to produce binocular vision.

Gas-permeable contact lens. A type of rigid contact lens that allows the passage of gases, the most important being oxygen, to nourish the cornea.

Glaucoma. An eye disease characterized by increased pressure within the eyeball.

  Absolute glaucoma. A final stage of untreated glaucoma that is generally characterized by blindness and eyes that are painful and chronically inflamed.

  Acute glaucoma. A type of glaucoma characterized by a sudden and severe increase in intraocular pressure. It generally causes pain, redness, and visual blur.

  Chronic glaucoma. The common type of asymptomatic glaucoma in which there is a slight and painless increase in intraocular pressure. *See also* Simple glaucoma; Secondary glaucoma.

  Closed-angle glaucoma. Another name for acute glaucoma.

  Congenital glaucoma. A type of glaucoma due to birth defects in the eye, it can occur at birth or in infancy.

  Low-tension glaucoma. A very rare type of glaucoma in which levels of intraocular pressure within the normal range cause glaucomatous changes.

  Open-angle glaucoma. Another name for chronic glaucoma.

  Secondary glaucoma. An increase in intraocular pressure caused by a known problem or medical disorder within the eyeball. For example, it can result from a previous eye infection. Both chronic and acute glaucoma can result from a secondary cause. *Compare* Simple glaucoma.

  Simple glaucoma. A type of chronic glaucoma in which the increase in intraocular pressure cannot be attributed to a known underlying cause. *Compare* Secondary glaucoma.

Glaucoma-suspect. In the absence of clinical glaucoma, a diagnosis in which some tests point to a tendency toward glaucoma, warranting more frequent than normal observation.

Gonioscope. An instrument equipped with prisms that can be placed on the cornea and will permit a clear view of the anterior drainage angle. It is of importance in the classification and treatment of glaucoma.

Graduated focal-length lens. A type of corrective glasses in which, from the top distance to the bottom reading correction, there is a range of intermediate focal distances. This is a new type of lens generally considered of limited use.

Gross visual field test. An examination of the visual field without specialized instrumentation, using only everyday objects like a pen or pencil.

Heat cautery. *See* Cyclodiathermy.

Hemorrhage. Bleeding; the seepage of blood from any type of blood vessel.

Herpes simplex. A virus that can infect the eye and sometimes cause dendritic ulcer.

Herpes zoster. A virus that can in rare cases infect the cornea or eyelids. The virus is also responsible for shingles and chicken pox.

Heterophoria. A condition in which there is an inward, outward, or upward tendency when the eyes are at rest. *See also* Esophoria; Exophoria; Hyperphoria.

Heterotropia. A condition in which there is an inward, outward, or upward deviation of one eye at rest or in use—that is, esotropia, exotropia, or hypertropia. It encompasses all types of strabismus.

Hordeolum. The common sty, an infection of a gland of the eyelid margin.

Hruby lens. A specialized lens that, when attached to the biomicroscope, permits visualization of the fundus.

Hydrophilic contact lens. The so-called soft contact lens, a type of contact lens made of plastic and capable of both absorbing and retaining water.

Hyperopia. The optical error in which an image has not yet come to a point of focus when it reaches the retina. Also called hypermetropia, it is commonly known as farsightedness.

Hyperphoria. A tendency of one eye to deviate upward when the eyes are at rest, it is a type of vertical eye muscle imbalance that can cause eye fatigue.

Hypertension. An increase above normal blood pressure levels, this condition can affect the eyes as well as the body as a whole.

Hypertensive retinopathy. A catchall term used to describe any of the various stages of retinal pathology caused by hypertension, including hemorrhages, thrombi, and papilledema.

Hypertropia. A type of strabismus in which there is an upward deviation of one eye in relation to the other when the eyes are at rest or in use.

Hyphema. A hemorrhage from the iris into the anterior chamber of the eye, frequently a result of trauma.

Hypopyon. The presence of a puslike fluid in the anterior chamber of the eye and secondary to an infection elsewhere in the eye.

Image size variation. A phenomenon caused by correction of anisometropia with eyeglasses, it can result in one eye seeing an image of a different size than that seen by the other eye.

Index of refraction. A measurement of the refractive power of a surface, how much that surface bends a ray of light passing through it.

Infectious conjunctivitis. An inflammation of the conjunctiva caused by a bacterial or viral infection.

Interstitial keratitis. An inflammation of the deeper layers of the cornea, producing clouding of the cornea. It is most frequently caused by syphilis or tuberculosis.

Intracapsular cataract extraction. A cataract extraction procedure in which the entire lens—capsule, cortex, and nucleus—is removed intact.

Intraocular pressure. The degree of firmness of the eyeball as controlled by secretion and drainage of aqueous fluid.

Iridectomy. A surgical procedure in which a portion of the iris is removed. It is frequently performed in glaucoma operations to facilitate drainage of aqueous fluid, and as part of cataract extractions to reduce the risk of secondary glaucoma.

Iridencleisis. A surgical procedure in which a section of the iris is pulled through the sclera to create a new drainage outlet for aqueous fluid. It is performed for certain cases of glaucoma.

Iris. A disclike diaphragm that is continuous with the ciliary body behind it and perforated in the center by the pupil. It is composed of vascular and muscular tissue, the latter controlling the size of the pupil. The color of the iris determines the color of an individual's eyes.

Iritis. Any inflammation of the iris.

Irregular astigmatism. An unusual type of astigmatism in which the unequal curvature of the cornea causes an image to be focused at more than two points along the visual axis.

Keratitis. Any inflammation of the cornea.

Keratoconjunctivitis. Any combined inflammation of the cornea and conjuctiva.

Keratoconus. A cone-shaped protrusion of the center of the cornea, it is caused by a progressive thinning of the corneal tissue layers due to a structural weakness. If it goes untreated, its effects are high, irregular astigmatism and eventual rupture of the cornea.

Keratometer. An optical instrument used to measure the curvature of the cornea, it is of particular use in the fitting of contact lenses.

Lacrimal apparatus. The system responsible for the formation, secretion, and drainage of tears, it includes the following:

> **Lacrimal canal:** A small channel along which tears drain from the punctum to the lacrimal sac.
>
> **Lacrimal duct:** The passageway through which tears are drained from the lacrimal sac into the back of the nose, and from there, into the throat.
>
> **Lacrimal fluid:** Tears.
>
> **Lacrimal gland:** The gland that manufactures the tears and is located in the upper, outer wall of the orbit.
>
> **Lacrimal lake:** The collection of tears in the conjunctival sac where the lower eyelid conjunctiva and scleral conjunctiva meet.
>
> **Lacrimal punctum:** A tiny elevation with a central hole located on the lower eyelid margin toward the nose. Its function is to siphon off the tears.
>
> **Lacrimal sac:** A small saclike pouch between the lacrimal canal and the lacrimal duct, it forms part of the tear drainage system.

Laser beam. A powerful, concentrated beam of light that

can generate a great deal of heat in a tiny, specified area. It can be used in glaucoma and retinal surgery.

Laser phakoablation. An experimental surgical procedure that would employ laser technology for cataract removal.

Lattice degeneration. A thinning of the retina in its far periphery, occuring in about 8 percent of the general population. It rarely causes a secondary retinal detachment and occurs most commonly in high myopia.

Lazy eye. *See* Amblyopia.

Legal blindness. Vision that cannot be corrected to better than 20/200, or the presence of extreme tunnel vision.

Lens (crystalline). A transparent and flexible body, convex on both surfaces and lying directly behind the iris of the eye. It serves to focus the rays of light on the retina.

Lens (optical). A transparent substance usually made of glass or plastic with two opposed surfaces, and used to bend light and thereby change the point at which light rays focus. It is used in the correction of optical errors.

Lensometer. An optical instrument used to determine the exact prescription of a pair of eyeglasses.

Light adaptation. The ability of the eye to adjust to bright illumination, this process occurs in the retina and entails an increase in the number of functioning cones and a decrease in the number of functioning rods. Complete light adaptation takes about one hour. *Compare* Dark adaptation.

Low-tension glaucoma. *See* Glaucoma.

Macula. The specialized central area of the retina responsible for sharp central vision. It surrounds the fovea centralis.

Malignant melanoma. A rare cancer that can originate in the choroid layer inside the eyeball.

Manifest refraction. The subjective portion of the refraction where the subject reports to the examiner which of two lenses provides superior vision. It is also known simply as manifest.

Meibomian gland. One of about 30 or 40 small glands near each eyelid that secrete a small amount of fatty lubricant at the eyelid margin to prevent normal amounts of tears from flowing over onto the cheek.

Metabolic cataract. An opacity of the lens of the eye caused by either a hormonal disorder (such as diabetes) or a biochemical disorder (such as a side effect of corticosteroid medication).

Microphthalmos. A condition in which the eyeball is abnormally small. It is usually a congenital condition.

Middle-distance vision. Use of the eyes to view objects in the area beyond arm's reach but within normal conversational distance. This is not a routinely measured ophthalmological distance, but in practical terms it is roughly a distance from two-and-a-half to five feet of the eyes. *Compare* Distance vision; Near Vision.

Miosis. Contraction of the pupil.

Miotic drops. A type of eyedrop causing contraction of the pupil and used therapeutically in the control of glaucoma.

Mixed astigmatism. A type of astigmatism in which one point of focus is in front of the retina and the other is theoretically behind the retina.

Monovision system. The use of contact lenses to correct

the symptoms of presbyopia together with myopia, or hyperopia, by providing one eye with the correction for near vision and the other the correction for distance vision. It relies on the phenomenon whereby the optic center of the brain selects the clearer image and suppresses the less-clear image.

Myopia. The optical error in which an object comes to a point of focus before it reaches the retina and is thus out of focus on the retina. It is commonly known as nearsightedness.

Nearsighted astigmatism. A type of astigmatism in which both points of focus are in front of the retina.

Nearsightedness. *See* Myopia.

Near vision. Ophthalmologically measured at 14 inches (33 centimeters), the normal reading distance. In practical terms, it is the vision used to view objects within arm's reach of the eyes, or up to about two feet. *Compare* Distance vision; Middle-distance vision.

Night blindness. Any of several rare eye diseases in which degeneration of specialized retinal tissue causes abnormally poor vision in dim light. *See also* Retinitis pigmentosa.

Noncontact applanation tonometry. A diagnostic test for glaucoma that involves flattening the cornea by applying pressure with an air pulse rather than touch. It is a means of measuring intraocular pressure.

Nonmedical contact lenses. Contact lenses used primarily for cosmetic and optical purposes, as opposed to those used to treat or control medical eye problems.

Normal vision. Two eyes with 20/20 visual acuity, fully developed binocularity, and normal peripheral vision.

Nucleus. The centermost portion of a structure. In the eye, the nucleus of the lens consists of the oldest cells; it is the part with the highest refractive function and the one that clouds most severely as senile cataracts form.

Nutritional cataract. A cataract caused by malnutrition that is seen in developing countries. It can also be an effect of anorexia nervosa or alcoholism.

Nystagmus. An involuntary, rhythmical oscillation of the eyeballs in a horizontal, vertical, or rotary direction. It may be caused by a central (neurological) problem or a localized eye problem, and can either cause or result from faulty visual development.

Objective test. A diagnostic test whose results are observed and determined by the tester rather than reported by the subject.

Ocular motility. The movement of the eyes, singly or together, laterally, vertically, obliquely, divergently, or convergently.

Oculist. Synonymous with ophthalmologist.

Oculo-kinetic perimetry. A visual field test in which the subject's eye, rather than the test stimulus, moves.

Open-angle glaucoma. *See* Glaucoma.

Ophthalmologist. A medical doctor trained in the diagnosis and treatment of eye diseases and correction of optical errors. An ophthalmologist is also known as an oculist.

Ophthalmoscope. An instrument equipped with a system of mirrors and lights with which the fundus of the eye can be examined.

Optic atrophy. Any condition in which the fibers of the optic nerve degenerate and finally die, causing corresponding loss of vision. Glaucoma is an example of optic atrophy.

Optic canal. The bony tunnel through which the optic

nerve runs from the back of the bony orbit into the front of the brain cavity.

Optic chiasm. An X-shaped area in the brain where the optic nerves of the right and left eyes meet and cross.

Optic disc. The portion of the optic nerve at the point of entrance into the back of the eye, it corresponds to the location of the blind spot.

Optic nerve. The nerve of sight, it is the collection of specialized nerve fibers derived from the retina that unite and send visual impulses to the brain.

Optic neuritis. Any inflammation of the optic nerve.

Optic tract. A specialized group of nerve fibers that begins in the optic chiasm and carries the visual impulses to the brain.

Optical error. *See* Ametropia.

Optical media. The transparent structures of the optical system through which light passes to focus an image on the retina. It includes the cornea, aqueous fluid, lens, and vitreous fluid.

Optician. A specialist who makes glasses in accordance with a doctor's prescription.

Optometrist. A doctor of optometry trained to test the eyes for nonmedical defects of vision in order to prescribe and dispense corrective lenses.

Ora serrata. The serrated edges located just behind the ciliary body that delineate the front ring of the retina and mark the limits of the retina's perceiving portion.

Orbit. *See* Bony orbit.

Orthophoria. The condition in which the two eyes are in perfect parallel alignment whether at rest or in use. It is therefore the completely normal balance of the eye-muscle functions.

Orthopic exercises. Training with eye exercises in an

attempt to improve eye-muscle balance. Such exercises are used effectively only occasionally and only in very young children.

Oxygen-permeable contact lens. *See* Contact lens.

Papilledema. A swelling of the optic disc that is usually caused either by interference with the blood circulation of the optic nerve through increased pressure from the brain cavity, by an inflammation of the optic nerve, or by hypertension.

Perimeter. An instrument that tests the peripheral visual fields as well as the blind spots of the eyes.

Peripheral iridectomy. The surgical removal of a minute portion of the iris at its root, this procedure is often performed as part of cataract extraction to lessen risk of secondary glaucoma by improving drainage of aqueous fluid.

Peripheral vision. Side vision, or the visual perception to all sides of the central object being viewed. It is vision other than central vision.

Peripheral visual field. *See* Visual fields.

Phakoemulsification. A cataract extraction technique in which the lens of the eye is sucked out through a needlelike probe.

Phoroptor. An instrument equipped with a broad selection of optical lenses that, when used singly or in combination, provide all possible optical corrections. This instrument is used primarily in testing the optics of the eye and in determining the prescription for corrective lenses.

Photorefractive keratectomy. An experimental procedure wherein a laser beam reshapes the cornea to theoretically reduce myopia.

Pingueculum. A fatty deposit that appears as a small,

raised, yellowish area on the horizontal midline of the sclera on either side of the cornea. It is nonpathological but can enlarge and become reddened, and has a greater tendency to appear in older people. A pingueculum does not interfere with vision.

Pinkeye. *See* Conjunctivitis.

Posterior chamber. The space behind the iris and in front of the lens that is filled with aqueous fluid. The aqueous is secreted into the posterior chamber and flows from there into the anterior chamber.

Presbyopia. The normal physiological change in the ability to focus on near objects, it occurs throughout life, normally becoming symptomatic in the 40s and resulting in total loss of ability to focus on near objects by around age 60. It normally requires correction with reading glasses in the mid-40s. The condition results from the increased inelasticity in the crystalline lens of the eye.

Prism. A transparent, solid structure with a triangular base used to disperse light into a color spectrum or to deflect rays of light toward the base of the triangle. It is used in eyeglasses to correct high degrees of extraocular muscle imbalance.

Progressive myopia. A lay term most commonly used in reference to the tendency of myopia to worsen during childhood growth.

Provocative tests for glaucoma. *See* Stress tests for glaucoma.

Pterygium. A triangular growth of thickened conjunctival tissue that usually extends from the portion of the conjunctiva nearest the nose to the border of the cornea or beyond, with its apex pointing toward the center of the cornea.

Ptosis. A drooping of the upper eyelid due to a congenital fault or to an acquired paralysis of the muscle that lifts the eyelid.

Pupil. The circular hole in the center of the iris.

Pupillary block. A condition in which normal circulation of aqueous fluid from the anterior to posterior chamber is mechanically impeded at the pupil, resulting in a severe and sudden rise in intraocular pressure.

Radial keratotomy. An experimental surgical procedure that attempts to correct optical defects with spokelike incisions in the cornea.

Refraction. The ophthalmological examination in which the nature and degree of optical errors present in the eye and the correction of these optical errors are determined. It also refers to the bending of a ray of light as it passes from air into a medium of greater optical density.

Refractive ability. The ability of an optical surface to bend light. *See also* Index of refraction.

Refractive surface. Any surface having the ability to bend light. *See also* Index of refraction.

Retina. The thin, delicate, transparent sheet of nerve tissue that lines the back two-thirds of the eyeball. It functions as the receptor of visual stimuli, which it transmits to the brain via the optic nerve.

Retinal detachment. A separation of the retina from the choroid.

Retinitis. Any inflammation of the retina.

Retinitis pigmentosa. A rare disease characterized by chronic and progressive degeneration of the retinal pigmentation. Hereditary in nature, it usually results in little or no vision by middle age. Night blindness is an early symptom.

Retinitis proliferans. A pathological condition characterized by a series of retinal hemorrhages, which in turn cause scar tissue to form on the retina and in the vitreous fluid. This will often result in severe visual loss and possible detachment of the retina. It is most commonly seen in diabetes.

Retinoblastoma. A rare malignancy originating in the retina. It often occurs in both eyes, and usually is found in very young children.

Retinoscope. An optical instrument that, through a system of mirrors and lights, is used to detect refractive errors in the eye.

Retrobubular neuritis. Any inflammation of the portion of the optic nerve lying behind the eyeball. It is generally accompanied by poor vision and is characteristically seen in connection with multiple sclerosis.

Retrolental fibroplasia. An abnormal growth of scar tissue in the vitreous fluid, accompanied by the abnormal growth of blood vessels, and retinal detachment. It is caused by the formerly common practice of administering high concentrations of oxygen to premature infants.

Rhodopsin. The pigment found in the rods of the retina, chemically important to dark adaptation. It is also known as visual purple.

Rods. Specialized cells of the retina sensitive to low intensities of light and important in dark adaptation.

Schiotz tonometry. A diagnostic test for glaucoma employing an instrument that measures the ease with which the cornea is indented. It is a means of determining intraocular pressure.

Sclera. The curved, opaque, protective white layer forming the back five-sixths of the outer coat of the eyeball. It is commonly known as the white of the eye.

Scleral buckling. A surgical eye procedure sometimes used in retinal detachment repair. The sclera is indented to create a groove, which in turn shortens the eyeball.

Scleral contact lens. A type of contact lens no longer in use that covered part of the sclera as well as the entire cornea.

Scleritis. Any inflammation of the sclera.

Scotoma. An abnormal area of varying size and shape within the visual field in which there is a partial or complete loss of vision.

Secondary cataract. A type of cataract caused either by a known condition of the eye or by a problem of general health other than simply advancing age. *See also* Cataract.

Senile cataract. The common type of cataract caused by advancing age. *See also* Cataract.

Single-vision lens. An optical lens having one focal length, or a lens in which there is only one optical correction.

Slit lamp. *See* Biomicroscope.

Snellen chart. The standard eye chart employed in the testing of distance visual acuity.

Sphincter pupillae. A circular muscle of the iris lying close to the pupillary margin. Its contraction causes constriction of the pupil and its relaxation causes dilation of the pupil. *Compare* Dilator pupillae.

Static perimetry. A visual field test that uses test stimuli at fixed positions, and in which luminance is gradually increased to the threshold of visibility.

Stereopsis. The visual perception of objects as three-dimensional rather than as all in one plane. Also known as depth perception.

Strabismus. A constant failure of the eyes to maintain parallel visual axes. It is commonly known as cross-eye.

Stress tests for glaucoma. A series of diagnostic tests that create a stress on the circulation of aqueous fluid within the eyeball and will increase intraocular pressure in an eye not healthy enough to withstand the stress. Used to assist in the diagnosis of glaucoma, the tests involve, in part, having a patient drink large quantities of fluid and sit in a dark room for a prolonged period of time in conjunction with a monitoring of intraocular pressure.

Sty. *See* Hordeolum.

Subconjunctival hemorrhage. The bleeding of a burst blood vessel that lies between the conjunctiva and sclera, resulting in a very red but painless eye.

Subjective test. A diagnostic test in which the results are reported by the test subject rather than observed by the tester.

Subluxation of the crystalline lens. A dislocation of the lens of the eye due to a rupture of the zonular attachment of the lens. The position the lens assumes depends on the location and extent of the rupture.

Sympathetic ophthalmia. An inflammation of the entire uveal tract of one eye invariably caused by a perforating wound that involves the uveal tissue of the other eye.

Synechia. Scar tissue extending from the iris, it most commonly follows an infection inside the eye and possibly causes secondary glaucoma or cataracts. It is known as *anterior synechia* if the scar tissue extends forward to the cornea and *posterior synechia* if the scar tissue extends backward to the lens.

Tangent screen. A flat, blackboardlike chart used in one type of test of the peripheral visual fields and blind spots of the eyes.

Thrombosis. The clotting of blood in any part of the circulatory system that blocks the passage of blood through the involved blood vessel.

Tonography. A test that can be performed as part of a glaucoma diagnostic workup, it monitors electronically the efficiency of the secretion/drainage mechanism inside the eye.

Tonometer. An instrument used to measure intraocular pressure, it is a principal part of diagnostic screening for glaucoma.

Tonometry. The diagnostic test performed with a tonometer.

Toric lens. A contact lens, both meridians of which are curved, but not to the same degree. It is designed to correct moderate to severe astigmatism.

Toxic conjunctivitis. *See* Chemical conjunctivitis.

Trabecular meshwork, network. A very fine fibrous, netlike tissue structure located in the recess of the anterior chamber, and through which aqueous fluid drains.

Trabeculectomy. A surgical procedure to treat glaucoma in which the drainage of aqueous fluid through the already existing drainage system is improved.

Trabeculoplasty. A surgical procedure to treat glaucoma that uses a laser beam to coagulate the trabecular meshwork and thus improve aqueous drainage.

Trabeculotomy. A surgical procedure to treat glaucoma

that opens a canal located in the trabecular meshwork in an attempt to improve aqueous drainage.

Trachoma. A contagious external eye infection. If it goes untreated, it may cause scarring of the cornea. It is a common cause of blindness in developing nations.

Traumatic cataract. An opacification of the lens caused by injury to it. Such a cataract can develop immediately or occur years after the injry. *See also* Cataract.

Trephine. A filtration procedure to improve aqueous drainage in the treatment of glaucoma. A disc of scleral tissue is removed, and aqueous fluid drains from the resulting hole into the subconjunctival space.

Trichiasis. An inversion of one or more of the eyelashes that causes friction resulting in irritation of the cornea or conjunctiva.

Trifocal lens. An eyeglass with three different optical portions, one for near vision, one for distance vision, and one for middle-distance vision.

20/20 vision. The expression of visual acuity indicating that the test subject can see at 20 feet what a normal-seeing subject can see at 20 feet. It is one of the components of normal vision. Also expressed as 6/6 to represent six meters rather than 20 feet.

Uveal tract. The vascular and muscular middle layer of the eyeball that consists of the iris, the ciliary body, and the choroid.

Uveitis. Any inflammation of the uveal tract.

Visual acuity. Sharpness of vision as determined by a comparison with the normal optical ability of an individual to define certain letters at a given distance, usually 20 feet. *See also* 20/20 vision.

Visual axis. The imaginary line extending from a viewed

object to the retina and passing through the air, corrective lenses (if any), cornea, aqueous fluid, pupil, crystalline lens, and vitreous fluid.

Visual field. The entire view encompassed by the eye when it is looking in a given direction, and the area visible to the eye, including sharp central and peripheral vision. It is also known as peripheral visual field.

Visual purple. *See* Rhodopsin.

Vitrectomy. Removal of vitreous fluid by suction and by cutting with an instrument that simultaneously replaces it with saline, another fluid, or other vitreous.

Vitreous floaters. *See* Floaters.

Vitreous fluid. A transparent, gel-like substance that fills the bulk of the interior of the eyeball, it begins behind the lens and attaches to the retina at the back and on the sides. It is also known as vitreous humor.

Vitreous implant. Surgical replacement of vitreous fluid following loss due to surgery or injury.

Xanthelasma. Cholesterol deposits that appear as yellowish, raised bumps on the surface of the skin on or near the upper and lower eyelids.

Zonule. The transparent membrane by which the crystalline lens is attached to the ciliary body.

Appendix

◇

Useful Addresses

American Academy of Ophthalmology
655 Beach Street
P.O. Box 7424
San Francisco, CA 94120-7424
Tel.: 415-561-8500
To obtain listing of board-certified ophthalmologists in
your area.

American Board of Medical Specialists
1 Rotary Center
Suite 805
Evanston, IL 60201
Tel.: 708-491-9091

The American Board of Ophthalmology
111 Presidential Boulevard
Suite 142
Bala Cynwyd, PA 19004
Tel.: 215-664-1175

Will give you a listing over the phone or by mail of board-certified ophthalmologists in your area.

Contact Lens Association of Ophthalmologists
523 Decatur Street
Suite 1
New Orleans, LA 70130
Tel.: 504-581-4000

A medical organization that will provide you with a list of medical contact-lens fitters in your area.

Index

Acetazolamide, 184–85
Acute glaucoma, 154–55, 168–69, 226
Acute secondary glaucoma, 155
Acute simple glaucoma, 155
Advertising by doctors, 270
Allergic conjunctivitis, 200
Allergic reactions, 245
Alternating-vision lenses, 80–81
American Academy of Ophthalmology,
    104, 237
American Association of Retired Persons
    (AARP), 242
Anterior chamber, 9
Anterior drainage angle, 150
Applanation tonometry, 157–60
Aqueous fluid, 9, 13–14, 150
Arteriosclerosis, 219–20
Artificial tears, 201, 240
Astigmatism, 43, 54–55
    contact lenses and, 60, 77–80
    eyeglass lens shape and, 70
    postoperative, 141, 145

Bacterial conjunctivitis, 198–99
Bifocal lenses
    contact, 80–81
    eyeglass, 63–67
    intraocular implants, 145
Biomicroscope, 32–34, 38, 158, 160
Bitoric lenses, 80
"Black eyes," 234
Bleeding. See Hemorrhaging
Blepharitis, 204
Blindness
    cataract-related, 107
    glaucoma-related, 147–48
Blind spot, 12–13
Blood supply to eyes, 10, 12
Bony orbit, 15
Brain, 17, 19–20, 47
B-scans, 268
"Buccaneer surgeons," 269–70
Burns, 203, 232–33, 235

Carbonic anhydrase inhibitors, 184
Cataract extraction, 112
Cataracts, 106–46
    case study, 116–38
    defined, 107
    diagnosis of, 115–22
    effects on vision, 107–108
    lens anatomy and, 108
    myths about, 106–107
    secondary, 111–12, 141–42, 144
    symptoms of, 109–10
    types of, 110–12
Cataract surgery, 113
    complications with, 138–42
    contact lenses and, 82–83, 123–25
    developments in, 142–46
    eyeglasses and, 137–38
    history of, 112
    implants, 123, 125–38, 141, 143–45
    indications for, 119–22
    local vs. general anesthesia for, 122–
        23
    myths about, 106, 114–15
    outpatient vs. hospital, 122
    pain from, 133–34
    postoperative care, 134–37
    preliminaries to, 127–28
    presurgery procedures, 128–29
    procedure, 129–33
    recommendation by ophthalmologist
        for, 125–26
    recovery, 133–34
    second opinions and, 126
Chalazions, 204–205
Chemical conjunctivitis, 200–201
Chemical eye injury, 227, 230–32
Chlamydia, 202
Choroid, 5, 9–10
Chronic secondary glaucoma, 154
Chronic simple glaucoma, 149, 153–54,
    171
Ciliary body, 5, 9, 15
Circulatory diseases, retina and, 218–22

Clip-ons, tinted, 256
Color-blindness, 196–97, 217–18
Computer users, eyeglasses for, 67–68
Concave lenses, 69–70
Cones, 12
Congenital cataracts, 110–11
Congenital glaucoma, 155–56
Conjunctiva, 5, 73–74
Conjunctivitis, 198–201
Consultation, 24–25, 41
Contact Lens Association of
    Ophthalmologists, 88
Contact lenses, 3, 70–103
    cataract surgery and, 123–25
    cleaning, 91–92, 95–96, 261–62
    cosmetic uses of, 82
    disposable, 86, 87
    economics of, 260–63
    extended-wear, 86–87
    vs. eyeglasses, 76–79
    eye makeup and, 248
    fitting of, 88–90
    hard, 71, 73, 75–76, 80, 83–84
    insertion of, 92–93, 96–97
    medical/optical uses of, 82–83
    myths about, 59–60
    nonmedical uses of, 79–81
    operation of, 73–76
    prescription of, 87–88
    removal of, 93–94, 97–98
    rigid gas-permeable. See Gas-
        permeable rigid contact lenses
    safety and, 70–71, 85, 91–98
    soft. See Soft contact lenses
    special problems, 98–103
    using, 90–98
Convex lenses, 70
Cornea, 5
    astigmatism and, 54–55
    burns of, 203, 235
    contact lenses and, 73, 83, 88, 90
    foreign particles on, 229, 235
    infections of, 202–203
    injuries to, 234–35
    metabolism of, 13, 73, 76
    passage of visual information
        through, 13, 18, 46–47
Cortisone, 200, 204
Cosmetic contact lenses, 82
Cosmetic eye surgery, 208–209
Cosmetics, 195, 245–48
Couching, 112
Cromolyn sodium, 200
Cryo-intracapsular cataract
    extraction, 143

Cryotherapy, 193–94, 213
Cupping, 159
Cyclodiathermy, 193–94, 213
Cystoid macular edema, 140
Cysts, retinal, 217

Dark adaptation, 12
Decentration of contact lenses, 100
Dentists, eyeglasses for, 68
Detached retina, 140, 212–15
Diabetes, 220–21
Diabetic retinopathy, 221
Dipivefrin, 181, 183
Discission surgery, 142
Discount optical houses, 251, 252
Diseases of the eye. See Eye diseases
Disposable contact lenses, 86, 87
Distance vision, 44–45
Diuretics, 184–85
Dry eyes, 208–209
Dyslexia, 196

Examination. See Eye examination
Examination room, 25–41
Expulsive choroidal hemorrhage, 139
Extended-wear contact lenses, 86–87
Extracapsular cataract extraction, 130–
    33, 142, 144
Eye care, 223–71
    choosing an eye doctor, 235–38
    contact lens economics, 260–63
    cosmetics, 195, 245–48
    eyeglasses. See Eyeglasses
    eyestrain, 248–49
    first aid, 225–35
    hazards of modern medicine to avoid,
        267–70
    health insurance, 264–66
    media and consumers, 270–71
    medications, 239–45
    myths about, 223–25
    proper lighting, 249–50
    second opinions, 126, 188, 225, 267
    visual training centers, 263–64
Eye cosmetics, 245–48
Eye diseases
    blepharitis, 204
    cataracts. See Cataracts
    chalazions, 204–205
    circulatory diseases and, 218–22
    color-blindness, 196–97, 217–18
    conjunctivitis, 198–201
    corneal infections, 202–203
    of external eye, 197–207
    eyelid tics, 207

glaucoma. *See* Glaucoma
myths about, 195–97
ptosis, 207
scleritis, 203
sties, 195, 201–202
subconjunctival hemorrhage, 206–207
vitreous floaters, 215
Eye doctors. *See* Ophthalmologists
Eyedrops
    administering, 242–44
    antiglaucoma, 181–83
    for blepharitis, 204
    for conjunctivitis, 200–201
    for corneal infections, 203
    diagnostic, 34–35
    generic vs. brand names, 241
    for red eyes, 239–40
Eye examination, 21–41
    age of child and, 224
    biomicroscope, 32–34, 38
    for cataracts, 116–22
    consultation, 24–25, 41
    contact lenses and, 90
    eyedrops, 34–35
    for glaucoma, 38–39, 148, 157–68, 171
    lensometer, 26–27
    myths about, 21–22
    need for, 23–24
    physical exam, 27
    refraction tests, 35–38
    retina check, 39–40
    Snellen Chart, 25–26
Eyeglass cases, 258
Eyeglasses, 58–70
    care and maintenance of, 257–60
    cataract surgery and, 137–38
    vs. contact lenses, 76–79
    defined, 62
    frames, 257–59
    history of use, 60–61
    myths about, 58–59
    need for, 61–62, 68
    purchasing, 251–57
    for special needs, 67–68, 260
    sunglasses, 59, 101–102, 255–57
    types of, 62–67
Eyeglass lenses
    bifocal, 63–67
    cleaning, 257–58
    glare-free coating, 254–55
    materials, 253–54
    scratched, 258
    shape of, 69–70

single-vision, 62–63
sunglasses, 255–56
tinted, 255
ultraviolet coating, 254–56
Eye infections, postoperative, 138
Eye injuries
    blows, 217
    first-aid for, 226–35
Eyelids, 15, 27, 232–33
Eyelid tics, 207
Eye makeup, 195, 245–48
Eye muscles
    farsightedness and, 51–52
    function of, 15–16
    presbyopia and, 56
    tests of, 27–28
Eye problems, common. *See* Optical errors
Eyes
    anatomy and function of, 4–13
    color of, 4, 8
    image recording and, 18–20
    myths about, 3–4
    passage of visual information through, 13
    structural prote   15–16
    visual process
Eyestrain, 52, 5
Eyewash, 223, 2

False eyelashes, 247
Farsightedness, 43, 50–54
    cataract surgery and, 123–24
    contact lenses and, 78, 79
    convex eyeglass lenses and, 70
    myths about, 42–43
Fibrillation, 207
Filtration procedures, 190–91
First aid, 225–35
Flat anterior chamber, 140
Fluorescein angiography, 210–11
Fluorescent lighting, 223–24, 250
Focusing, 9
Foldable lens implants, 144
Foreign particles in the eye, 227–30, 235
Frames, eyeglass, 257–59
Fundus photography, 167, 211

Gas-permeable rigid contact lenses, 76, 84–89
    astigmatism and, 80
    cleaning, 91–92
    fitting of, 88–89
    insertion of, 92–93

Gas-permeable rigid contact lenses (cont'd)
    prescription of, 87–88
    removal of, 93–94
    vs. soft contact lenses, 72–73, 84–86
Gels, antiglaucoma, 183–84
Generic medications, 241
Glare, 101–102
Glare-free coating, 254–55
Glasses. See Eyeglasses
Glaucoma, 147–94
    acute, 154–55, 168–69, 226
    case studies, 172–80, 185–91
    chronic simple, 149, 153–54, 171
    defined, 148–50
    diagnosis, 157, 168, 172–75
    effects of, 150–53
    emergencies, 168–69
    eye examinations for, 148
    medications for, 181–85
    myths about, 147, 170–71
    postsurgical management, 194
    routine testing, 38–39, 148, 157–60
    secondary to cataract surgery, 139–40
    specialized testing, 160–68
    surgery for, 185–94, 269
    treatment of, 175–94
    types of, 153–57
Glaucoma-suspect group, 168
Gonioscopy, 161–62
Gross visual field test, 33–34

Hard contact lenses, 71, 73, 75–76, 80,
    83–84
Health insurance, 264–66
Health Maintenance Organizations
    (HMOs), 265–66
Hemorrhaging
    first-aid for, 227
    postoperative, 139
    retinal, 215–16
    subconjunctival, 206–207
Herpes, 195, 202
High blood pressure. See Hypertension
Hruby lens, 160
Hyperindex 160 plastic lenses, 254
Hyperopia. See Farsightedness
Hypertension, 127, 147, 220

Implants, lens, 123, 125–38, 141, 143–
    45
Infections
    contaminated medication containers
        and, 244–45
    corneal, 202–203

postoperative, 138
    retinal, 216–17
Infectious conjunctivitis, 198–99
Insurance
    contact lens, 262–63
    health, 264–66
Intraocular inflammation, 139
Intraocular lens implants, 123, 125–38,
    141, 143–44
Intravenous antiglaucoma medication,
    185
Iridectomy, 191
Iridencleisis, 193
Iris, 5–7, 18

Keratoconus, 83
Keratometer, 88
Knife surgery, for glaucoma, 192–93

Lacrimal gland, 13
Laser phakoablation, 145
Laser scanning, preventive, 145–46
Laser surgery
    for detached retina, 213–14
    for glaucoma, 187–92, 269
    unnecessary, 269
Lattice degeneration, 140
Lenses
    bifocal. See Bifocal lenses
    contact. See Contact lenses
    eyeglass. See Eyeglass lenses
    intraocular implants, 123, 125–38,
        141, 143–45
    single-vision, 62–63
Lens of eye, 9, 13–15, 47, 108
Lensometer, 26–27
Light adaptation, 12
Lighting
    myths about, 223
    proper, 249–50
Low-tension glaucoma, 156–57

Macula, 11–13, 19
Macular degeneration, 221–22
Makeup, 195, 245–48
Media, unproven technologies and,
    270–71
Medicare, 266
Medications, 239–45
Middle distance vision, 45–46
Monovision system, 81
Muscles. See Eye muscles
Musicians, eyeglasses for, 68
Myopia. See Nearsightedness

Near-focusing muscles, 51–52, 55, 56
Nearsightedness, 43, 46–51
 cataracts and, 106
 convex eyeglass lenses and, 69–70
 eyeglasses vs. contact lenses and, 76–77
 myths about, 42–43
Near vision, 44–45
Newborn babies, 3, 17
Night blindness, 197
Noncontact applanation, 159
Normal vision, 44
Nucleus, 108
Nutritional cataracts, 111

Oculists. See Ophthalmologists
Oculo-kinetic perimetry, 167
Ointments
 administering, 242–44
 antiglaucoma, 183–84
Ophthalmologists, 235–38
 at clinics, 235
 contact lenses and, 87, 88, 260–61
 ethics and, 267–70
 examination by. See Eye examination
 fees of, 238
 finding, 237–38
 vs. opticians, 224
 vs. optometrists, 115, 224, 236–37
 second opinions and, 267
 specialists vs. generalists, 238
Ophthalmoscope, 39–40, 159–60, 210
Optical errors, 42–57
 correction of. See Contact lenses;
  Eyeglasses; Radial keratotomy
 myths about, 42–43
 vs. normal vision, 44
 types of. See Astigmatism;
  Farsightedness; Nearsightedness;
  Presbyopia
 vision measurement and, 44–46
Optical media, 13
Optic disc, 151, 159–60, 164, 167
Opticians, 224, 251–53
Optic nerve, 5, 8, 12–13, 19, 151, 159–60, 164
Optometrists, 87, 115, 224, 236–37, 252
Oral antiglaucoma medications, 184–85
Oval discs, antiglaucoma, 183, 184

Pain, from cataract surgery, 133–34
Patient history, 24–25
Penetrating eye injury, 226–27

Perimeters, 165–67
Peripheral iridectomy, 131
Phakoemulsification, 115, 143
Phoroptor, 36
Photorefractive keratotomy, 49
Physical exam, 27
Pigment epithelial detachment, 221
Pilocarpine, 181
Pinkeye, 198–201
Plastic lenses, 253–54
Plastic surgery, 208–209
Polycarbon plastic lenses, 254, 260
Posterior chamber, 9
Preadmission tests, 127
Presbyopia, 43, 56–57, 69–70
Prescription drugs, 241–42
Preventive laser scanning, 145–46
Private health insurance, 264–65
Progressive myopia, 50
Ptosis, 207
Pupil, 5
Pupillary block, 139–40

Radial keratotomy, 49, 103–105
Reading glasses, ready-made, 253
Red eyes, 239–41
Refraction tests, 35–38
Refractive ability, 47
Retina
 anatomy of, 10–11
 disorders of, 209–22
 farsightedness and, 50–51
 function of, 11–12
 image recording and, 18–20
 nearsightedness and, 47
 visual process and, 17
Retina check, 39–40
Retinal detachment, 140, 212–15
Retinitis pigmentosa, 197
Retinoscope, 36–37
Ridley, Harold, 143–44
Rigid contact lenses
 chipped and scratched, 98–99
 cleaning, 91–92
 gas-permeable. See Gas-permeable
  rigid contact lenses
 hard, 71, 73, 75–76, 80, 83–84
 insertion of, 92–93
 removal of, 93–94
 replacement of, 99
Rods, 12

Schiotz tonometry, 157–58, 160
Sclera, 5, 151

Scleritis, 203
Secondary cataracts, 111–12, 141–42, 144
Secondary glaucoma, 139–40, 154, 155
Second opinions, 126, 188, 225, 267
Senile cataracts, 110
Simultaneous-vision lenses, 80–81
Single-vision lenses, 62–63
Snellen Chart, 25–26
Soft contact lenses, 71–72, 76
    cleaning, 95–96, 261–62
    fitting of, 89–90
    vs. gas-permeable contact lenses, 72–73, 84–86
    insertion of, 96–97
    prescription of, 87
    removal of, 97–98
    replacement of, 99
Static perimetry, 166–67
Sties, 195, 201–202
Strabismus, 30, 196
Stress test, 162–63
Structural protection, 15–16
Subconjunctival hemorrhage, 206–207
Sunglasses, 59, 101–102, 255–57
Surgery
    for cataracts. See Cataract surgery
    cosmetic, 208–209
    for detached retina, 212–14
    for glaucoma, 185–94, 269
    laser. See Laser surgery
    unnecessary, 268–69

Tangent screen, 164–65
Tears, 13
Tests, unnecessary, 267–68
Three-dimensional vision, 18–19, 31
Tics, eyelid, 207

Timolol maleate, 181, 183
Tinted glasses, 59
Tonography, 163
Tonometers, 38–39, 157–59
Toric lenses, 80
Toxic conjunctivitis, 200–201
Trabecular meshwork, 174, 191
Trabeculectomy, 191
Trabeculoplasty, 191
Trabeculotomy, 191
Trephine, 193
Trifocals, 66, 67
Tumors, retinal, 217
20/20 vision, 44, 50, 59

Ultraviolet coating, 254–56
Ultraviolet radiation, 233
Uveal tract, 5

Viral conjunctivitis, 198–99
Vision, 13–20
    distance, 44
    middle distance, 45–46
    near, 44–45
    normal, 44
Visual axis, 13
Visual field tests, 164–67, 211–12
Visual information, passage of, 13–15
Visual process, 16–20
Visual training centers, 263–64
Vitamin A, 196, 240–41
Vitrectomy, 214
Vitreous floaters, 215
Vitreous fluid, 13, 15, 18
Vitreous implant, 214

Zonule, 9